Visual display units:
Job content and stress in office work

Visual display units: Job content and stress in office work

New technologies and the improvement
of data-entry work

FE JOSEFINA F. DY

INTERNATIONAL LABOUR OFFICE   GENEVA

ISBN 92-2-105083-1 (limp cover)
ISBN 92-2-105084-X (hard cover)

First published 1985

Cover photograph: ILO Photo Library/J. Maillard

Printed in Switzerland   IRL

FOREWORD

The rapid spread of new technology is bringing about substantial changes in the nature of office work. Some people have high expectations of this transformation, while others foresee negative effects on workers and work organisation. It is certainly true to say that office automation offers both opportunities and constraints. The ILO has always maintained a keen interest in the particular needs of office workers, and all the more so at the present time, when such work is undergoing change, and when the number of workers affected is rapidly expanding.

This book explores a common office task—that of the data-entry operator working on a visual display unit or keypunch. It first presents a brief historical survey of the development of data-entry work, and then goes on to cover the various aspects of such jobs today: work organisation and working time; health, safety and ergonomics; and occupational stress. By carefully examining both the technological and the organisational options which are available, and by analysing in depth the conditions associated with some of these options, it is demonstrated that serious problems—both in physical and psychological terms—exist for many data-entry workers. Finally, the book attempts to show that choices are available, as regards work design and working conditions, which prevent these problems from occurring or at least mitigate their effects.

The book is aimed at consultants, managers, trade unionists, workers and other individuals affected by new office technology. It is hoped that they will find it a useful tool in planning and introducing data-entry jobs which are more satisfying and rewarding to all concerned.

CONTENTS

Figures

Acknowledgements

For permission to reproduce copyright material, grateful acknowledgement is due to the following: Dartnell Corporation, Chicago (example 1, p. 17); John Wiley and Sons, New York and Chichester, United Kingdom (example 2, p. 18); Christine Davis and Online Publications, Uxbridge, United Kingdom (example 3, p. 19); CLC Educational Services (formerly CLC Labour Education and Studies Centre), Ottawa (figure 1, p. 43); Thomas Nelson and Sons, Walton-on-Thames, United Kingdom (figure 2, p. 95)

Abbreviations

ANACT	Agence nationale pour l'amélioration des conditions de travail (France)
BLS	Bureau of Labor Statistics (United States)
CHD	coronary heart disease
CLC	Canadian Labor Congress

CRT   cathode ray tube
EDP   electronic data processing
EEC   European Economic Community
FIET   International Federation of Commercial, Clerical and Technical Employees
MICR   magnetic ink character recognition
MT/ST   Magnetic Tape Selectric Typewriter
NIOSH   National Institute for Occupational Safety and Health (United States)
OCR   optical character recognition
OMR   optical mark recognition
RF   radio frequency
TUC   Trades Union Congress (United Kingdom)
VDT   visual display terminal
VDU   visual display unit

INTRODUCTION

"Office automation", "the electronic office" or "the office of the future" are phrases frequently heard today. A microprocessor-driven wave of technological innovation is having pervasive effects on a sector which has traditionally been labour intensive and virtually bereft of significant technological change. Yet some electronic offices or offices of the future are said to exist already, some are in the prototype phase and others are being planned. New options are being developed and many more are expected in the future.

The technologies of the electronic office include word processing, electronic mail and filing systems, advanced reprographics, facsimile transmission, "smart" copiers and "intelligent" telephones. Office employees, both management and workers, are confronted by new work systems, new communication patterns, new organisational structures and new skills. These changes, perhaps more than the technological advances, are affecting the jobs people do, their position in the organisational system and their relationships with each other. Thus the introduction of new technologies influences workers' responsibilities, skill requirements, job content, physical and mental workload, career prospects and social relationships at work.

While technological change is inevitable, the challenge facing managers, trade union representatives and individuals is how to take advantage of the opportunities offered by new technology to redesign and restructure jobs so that they are made more interesting and more satisfying, rather than more monotonous, more stressful or more frustrating. This is not an easy task. It will require considerable planning, skill and goodwill.

A step in the right direction is that the electronic office has become a subject of public discussion. Governments, management, trade unions and individual workers are showing increasing interest in the problems and the potential of the electronic office. Moreover, most experts agree that technological limitations to the development of the electronic office are minor compared with the difficulties of overcoming organisational and individual resistance. This in itself is forcing manufacturers and technology experts to come to terms with the "human factor" of the electronic office.

The electronic office promises an array of benefits. For some office workers, it can result in the elimination of the repetitive and more tedious aspects of their jobs. This means not only more varied and interesting work but also, in certain circumstances, additional responsibilities and the opening of new career opportunities. For example, a secretary who is not retyping a report for the third time can be doing other work which is potentially more interesting. One of the frequently mentioned advantages of the electronic office is that it minimises, if not eliminates, retyping, sorting, filing and message taking. Moreover, the powerful capabilities of word-processing technology increase the skill requirements of the typing job where the typist has to visualise, design and amend the presentation of a text. Computer capabilities also provide rapid access to information, which enables the office worker to respond directly to the needs of clients and customers. This, in turn, gives the worker opportunities for decision-making, problem-solving and control over the job.

While the status of general clerks has declined, the relatively new occupations associated with the transfer of clerical work to computers (i.e. systems designers and computer programmers) have attracted higher status. As more new office technologies with sophisticated software become available, the increased simplicity of programming computers may facilitate the transfer back to clerical workers of some discretion and autonomy on the job.

The electronic office is attractive primarily for economic reasons. The rapidly falling cost of equipment in real terms, together with its increased capacity to store and manipulate large volumes of information rapidly and accurately, will more and more influence decisions towards investments in the electronic office. Moreover, the need to increase productivity and to reduce escalating labour costs is becoming more urgent to management.

While the electronic office offers opportunities, it also poses problems.

The employment implications of the electronic office are major issues of concern. Increasing evidence shows that the extra efficiency of new technology can often lead to job losses. Many trade unions are naturally disturbed at the negative effects both for their own members and for overall employment levels.

Whatever the quantitative impact on employment levels, however, the electronic office has also been associated with negative effects on the content and organisation of work. Some workers find that the electronic office "deskills" those jobs that remain. By allocating as much content as possible to the technology, jobs are reduced to minimum skills. Once the novelty of new equipment has worn off, workers find that unsatisfying, repetitive, menial tasks have been replaced by new tasks with as little or even less interest and status. By taking away the most interesting parts of the job, the electronic office can devalue or render irrelevant hard-learnt skills. Some workers complain of being isolated in "data centres" where pay is low and career opportunities seem few.

The electronic office can not only streamline office operations but can also expand managerial supervision significantly. Many workers resent loss of control over their own jobs, particularly when the computer monitors their performance and prompts them on what to do next. Many complain of increased workload, work intensity and high levels of stress, eye-strain and other hazards. As an editorial in *Computerworld* states—

Hardly a day passes that a reader of general-interest newspapers and magazines does not see a story about a computer foul-up or about computerisation's dehumanising effect on the work environment. Unfortunately, many of these stories are true. Often systems are installed with little regard for the worker—especially if a project ends up exceeding budget.[1]

Thus, while the electronic office holds enormous potential to improve the content of jobs and working conditions, the reverse can also occur. The electronic office can help to initiate, reinforce or perpetuate management systems, work methods and working conditions which have negative effects on office workers. Much depends on the choices made concerning how new technology will be used and how it will be introduced. New office technology is very flexible, but it must be applied in appropriate ways if its potential is to be realised.

FOCUS OF THE STUDY

This study is about data-entry work. Specifically, it looks at two main data-entry jobs influenced by computerisation: keypunch jobs and word-processing jobs. The main function of these jobs is to encode alphanumeric[2] data by hitting the keys of a keyboard.

In order to understand the nature of data-entry jobs, it is necessary to make a distinction between encoding alphanumeric data on a full-time basis and doing it as part of a job. Data encoding is a task: it can be combined with other tasks to make a job, or can in itself be the job when it is the only activity performed. For example, a secretarial job can include the tasks of stenography, filing, typing, handling mail, arranging appointments, etc., while a typist in a typing pool only has one task, that of keying or typing. Similarly, there is a distinction between using a machine occasionally as an adjunct or aid and using it full time. Workers who use the machine full time resemble machine operators.

Some of the problems of data-entry workers were already well known in the 1960s, when keypunch operators were studied. Their jobs were seen to be simplified, narrow and demanding, while requiring both accuracy and speed. The workers were deprived of freedom of movement about the office, interaction with co-workers and opportunities for advancement. Keypunch jobs were found to be analogous to assembly-line jobs. Significantly, managers noting the results of these early studies ignored the ill effects reported. They asserted that eventually technological advances would render this mode of data entry obsolete.[3]

Today the problems still exist. Although computer technology has changed rapidly, the vast majority of computer input is still supplied by key-driven alphanumeric devices. The data preparation technologies of the electronic office are merely adding new dimensions to already familiar problems. The principal difference lies in the ever larger number of workers involved. The similarity is that the workers who hold these jobs are mostly women and that they are usually at the lower levels of the organisational hierarchy.

METHODOLOGICAL APPROACH

This study concentrates on the potential for improving the quality of working life of data-entry workers.

"Quality of working life" is a comprehensive popular term which focuses on job-related factors in the overall quality of life. It is a multidimensional concept which subsumes the characteristics of the job itself, the working environment and conditions of employment. It also includes the various ways in which workers can make decisions concerning the design and performance of their jobs, as well as their reactions and attitudes.

While the data-entry technology, tasks and the way these tasks are organised into data-entry jobs are important, it is also necessary to consider the workers who carry out these tasks and fill these jobs: their age, sex, educational background and experience; their expectations, attitudes and preferences about work; and the effects that their work has on them. These individual characteristics and differences are critical in analysing the relationship between each individual and her[4] work.

The major theme of this study is that there are organisational choices concerning data-entry work which could improve the quality of working life and conditions of work without sacrificing organisational effectiveness. There are, however, constraints on these choices: these constraints may be organisational, technological and social.

For example, whether data-entry tasks are assigned to specialist groups or individuals or distributed among a larger group of workers depends upon organisational structures and procedures. In many cases, there are alternative structures and procedures for getting the same work done. In order to illustrate such options, three possible configurations are considered as examples. In one example, a number of data-entry jobs are centralised in a word-processing centre. In a second example, the same data-entry work is assigned to separate administrative units where the data-entry workers continue to work full time encoding data. Finally, the data-entry work is shared among a larger group of workers so that no one has a full-time data-entry job.

While the above examples illustrate possibilities, there are constraints which may make certain options impractical or difficult. A first set of constraints relates to the difficulty of changing existing hardware, procedures and programmes, organisational patterns or individual duties. For example, moving from the first to the third organisational configuration (centralised to decentralised data entry) previously described would usually require physically moving and rewiring the data-entry hardware or acquiring more terminals and printers, changing the work flow and retraining a number of workers. In some cases, these difficulties in making changes exist even when new technologies are being introduced, and should be considered as a potential for change: for example, the existence of a typing pool can lead to a decision to install a word-processing centre in order to retain the existing organisational structure.

A second kind of constraint relates to the amount of data entry in the overall work carried out in a particular office or work setting. If the proportion of data-entry work is extremely high, there will need to be at least some jobs with close to full-time data entry; if the proportion is low, it is easier to share out the work and make it a small part of many jobs. However, these constraints could be overcome if the social and technical implications of new technology were considered in its design and introduction. The current state of the technology makes it quite feasible to include design specifications which lead to more satisfying work.

In Chapter 1, data-entry work is examined from a historical and sociological viewpoint. Data-entry tasks, jobs and equipment are also described. The chapter concludes with a brief discussion concerning the extent and future trend of data-entry work.

In Chapter 2, the implications of computerisation for work organisation and working time are discussed.

Chapter 3 considers an area which has been the focus of much attention during the last few years: the health, safety and ergonomic aspects of data-entry workplaces.

Chapter 4 focuses on occupational stress. Stress is one of the major complaints of clerical workers using computer-based technologies and has been shown to be related to various diseases and psychological disorders.

Chapter 5, on the potential to improve data-entry jobs, presents a number of practical suggestions based on the organisational and technological choices which have been shown to exist. It emphasises measures which can be expected to improve the quality of working life of the workers concerned, while paying due attention to organisational effectiveness. The roles of governments, employers and trade unions in implementing these measures are also discussed.

Notes

[1] "Regard for the worker", editorial in *Computerworld* (Framingham, Massachusetts), 24 Mar. 1980, p. 20.

[2] Alphanumeric: data or text containing both the letters of the alphabet and the numerals 0–9.

[3] See, for example, Ida Russakoff Hoos: "The impact of office automation on workers", in *International Labour Review* (Geneva, ILO), Oct. 1960, pp. 363–388; idem "When the computer takes over the office", in *Harvard Business Review* (Boston), July–Aug. 1960, pp. 102–112; James C. Taylor: *Fragmented office jobs and the computer* (Geneva, ILO, 1978; mimeographed internal working document; restricted).

[4] As previously mentioned, almost all data-entry workers are women. The pronouns "she" and "her" are therefore used in this study.

THE CHANGING NATURE OF OFFICE WORK

1

ORIGINS AND CONTEXT OF DATA-ENTRY WORK

In order to appreciate the impact of new technology on conditions of work and quality of working life of data-entry workers, it is helpful to look at office work from a historical and sociological perspective.

Office work in its early stages has been likened to a craft.[1] Early offices were small, as were the businesses they serviced. They were staffed almost exclusively by men. These office workers—who were then called "clerks"—were "all-round" workers: in other words, they handled all aspects of their assignment. In many ways, these office workers had responsibilities which would nowadays be classified as "managerial".

The small size of offices also meant that the relationship between employer and clerk tended to be very personalised. The clerks worked under the direct supervision, and often the direct view, of their employers. Although they were generally given well-defined jobs, they had a certain amount of discretion in carrying them out. Moreover, they were often asked to do numerous different tasks by their employers.

Traditionally, office workers had better working conditions than many other categories of worker. They enjoyed shorter and more convenient hours than factory workers. They worked in clean surroundings, and in terms of functions, authority, pay, tenure of employment (a clerical position was usually a lifetime post), career prospects, status and even dress, an office worker was undeniably middle class, a professional, a skilled craftsman and a part of management.[2]

The last decades of the nineteenth and the first decades of the twentieth centuries marked the rise of modern industrial capitalism and the growth in scope and size of organisations. As business operations became larger and more complex, there was a corresponding increase in the volume of communication, record-keeping and office work in general. This period of expansion marked the growth of bureaucracy, and a system of work organisation which attempted to maintain overall control and co-ordination of larger and more complex organisations, which posed increasingly difficult problems for business. Bureaucracy is also characterised by the substitution of informal groupings by formal organisations.

7

According to Weber, bureaucratic structures contain the following major characteristics: a continuous organisation of official functions bound by rules (standardisation); a specific sphere of competence (specialisation); and each lower office under the control and supervision of a higher one (hierarchy).[3]

With the enormous changes in scale and the growth of bureaucracy, the texture and shape of office work were also altered. Personalised work relationships and the atmosphere of mutual obligation were replaced by impersonal and standardised relationships as the office moved from small and only partially structured groupings to much larger, highly structured aggregations. The status of clerical work in society also changed. Clerical workers were no longer a few quasi-managerial, relatively high-status employees; they were a large occupational category. Moreover, economic status deteriorated for most categories of office worker as the income gap between manual and non-manual work narrowed substantially. This occupational category included a growing proportion of women, with the result that clerical work gradually became a female occupation.

These changes also marked the transformation of the office hierarchy. A new male managerial stratum took over the quasi-managerial activities of the clerks, leaving the detailed, routine work to the new, predominantly female staff. Two distinct occupational hierarchies evolved: a male one, made up of several layers of managers, and a female one of filing clerks, typists, stenographers, clerical supervisors and secretaries. This marked the beginning of the increasing distinction in clerical or office work between those conceptualising the task (mental work) and those carrying it out (manual work).

The rise of middle-level managers, who became the dominant group in the office, and the feminisation of clerical work fundamentally altered the meaning and prestige of clerical work. More and more, clerical work meant the carrying out of routine tasks, planned, set up and supervised by others. A clerical job was viewed less and less as a stepping-stone to management and business success. A survey conducted in the late 1920s showed that 88 per cent of the office managers "felt they needed clerks who were satisfied to remain clerks".[4] Thus, women entered the workforce in occupations that no longer offered the traditional advantages of white-collar jobs; they found themselves in occupations that were declining in social and economic status.

The rationalisation of office work: scientific management

The division of labour brought about by increased organisational size and bureaucracy coincided with the scientific management movement which culminated in the work of F. W. Taylor.[5] In view of its continued prevalence (with implicit or explicit application) and its far-reaching implications for work design and job content, it is important to review briefly the characteristics of scientific management.

"Scientific management" was originally used to analyse and eventually control the work process in the factory. As the name implies, it represents an attempt to use a scientific and systematic approach to managerial decision-making. Scientific management, according to Taylor's formulations, is characterised by the separation of conception from execution of tasks (distinction between mental and manual labour); task specialisation and standardisation through the application of work study; the selection of the "first-class man" for every specific task; and motivation of the worker through compensation—specifically, the differential piece-rate system ("a fair day's pay for a fair day's work").

Taylor's principles were based on his diagnosis of the existing industrial situation and can be reduced to one simple theme: inefficiency. One of the methods that Taylor emphasised to reduce inefficiency was the design and planning of work by specialised "scientific managers". "All possible brainwork should be removed from the shop and centred in the planning or laying-out department . . .".[6] This meant that the worker did not participate in the planning of his work. His tools, work methods, procedures, and so on, were "scientifically" designed for him to ensure order, efficiency and machine-like synchronisation of work flows.

In addition to his principle of separation between conception and execution, Taylor advocated that each worker be assigned each day a specific amount of work, of a certain quality based on the results of time study. This assigned quota he called a "task". In *The principles of scientific management*, Taylor pointed out that—

The work of every workman is fully planned out by the management at least one day in advance, and each man receives in most cases complete instructions, describing in detail the task which he is to accomplish, as well as the means to be used in doing the work. . . . This task specifies not only what is to be done, but how it is to be done and the exact time allowed for doing it.[7]

Taylor aimed to relate to each other in "the best way" the methods adopted, the time taken, the tools used and the fatigue generated by any task.

Taylor's prescriptions concerning selection, training and motivation were also based on his two previous principles. Selection of the "first-class man" was based solely on the ability of the worker to perform the tasks as specified by time and motion studies. Training implied seeing to it that the worker had a complete grasp of the routine movements of a given task and that he maintained the specified level of speed and efficiency. One prerequisite of successful training was also to convince the worker that he could not know better than the scientific manager how a job should be done.

Motivation, according to Taylor, was directly, if not solely, related to the compensation system. Taylor asserted that the definition of "a fair day's work" was a purely technical matter determined by production engineers after work study. On the other hand, a definition of "a fair day's pay" was more elusive, though Taylor believed that it should be substantially above the rate for similar kinds of work in the locality. Its critical feature, however, was that the level of reward should be closely tied to output, through the mechanism of the differential piece-rate system. Accordingly, a worker who failed to produce "a fair day's work" should suffer a proportionate loss of earnings; and, if he excelled the target, he should receive a bonus.

Although initially meant for the factory, scientific management rapidly invaded the office—

Time and motion study reveal just as startling results in the ordinary details of clerical work as they do in the factory. And after all, since every motion of the hand and body, every thought, no matter how simple, involves the consumption of physical energy, why should not the study and analysis of these motions result in the discovery of a mass of useless effort in clerical work just as it does in the factory?[8]

Thus writes William Henry Leffingwell, in 1917, in his book entitled *Scientific office management*, and subtitled *A report on the results of applications of the Taylor system of scientific management to offices, supplemented with a discussion of how to obtain the most of these results.*

Earlier Charles Babbage, who designed one of the first calculating engines ("computers"), discussed the possibility of separating conception and execution in mental labour in his book *On the economy of machinery and manufactures*, written in the 1830s.[9] In a prophetic chapter entitled "On the division of mental labour", he suggested that the division of labour could be applied with equal success to mental as to mechanical operations, and that it might produce the same savings in time. He used as an example the division of labour among three groups or sections of people given the task of adapting mathematical tables to the decimal system during the French Revolution. The first group consisted of five or six eminent French mathematicians who designed the formulae to be used by the other sections. The second group, made up of seven or eight people with a good knowledge of mathematics, was to convert these formulae into numerical values and to devise means of checking the calculations. The third group, varying in number between 60 and 80 persons, did nothing more than simple addition and subtraction and returned the results to the second group for checking. Babbage was astonished to discover that, although nine-tenths of those in the third group had no knowledge of arithmetic apart from the first two rules that they were called upon to use, they were usually found to be more correct in their calculations than those who had a more extensive knowledge of the subject.

Two conclusions may be drawn from Babbage's work: first, the labour of educated or better-paid persons should not be "wasted" on matters that can easily be done by those with lesser training; and second, those with little or no training are superior in the performance of routine work because they are undistracted by too much mental effort, and their work is "mechanical". In addition, according to Babbage, they can be employed at a low wage.

Babbage also foresaw the time when the "calculating engine" would eliminate the operations of addition and subtraction performed by the third group, and then eventually the work of the second group. He envisaged the transformation of the whole process into mechanical routine supervised by the first group, which would be the only one required to understand the mathematics involved or the process itself. The work of the others would be converted into the preparation of data and the operation of machinery.

As long as offices were small and white-collar workers were a genteel minority in relation to production workers, clerical workers were more or less self-supervising and relatively immune from too rigorous cost-benefit analysis. However, as offices expanded, the need to make clerical work more efficient gained importance. Under scientific management, decision-making on how work should be carried out became centralised in the hands of the office manager. In 1918, Lee Galloway published his standard work, *Office management: Its principles and practice*, which emphasised that "it is the work of the office organisation, under the supervision of the office manager, to devise records, methods and systems for carrying out the function of control and for co-ordinating the activities of one department with those of another".[10]

To "streamline" and "rationalise" the office, the early practitioners of scientific management atomised, standardised and regulated office work. Elaborate studies were carried out on all forms of clerical work, not only on those which were already routine and repetitive. Stenographic and typing output were rigorously scrutinised. Some typewriter companies even equipped their machines with a mechanical contrivance which automatically counted the strokes made on the typewriter and recorded them on a dial. This meter was used together with a time-clock which the typist punched at the beginning and end of each job. Metering of this kind was used as the basis for piece-work payments.

Dictation time was also recorded, at first by page and later, with the spread of dictating machines, by mechanical means. Daily records of the amount of work performed by each clerk were kept in order to know her "capacity" and to spur her "to even better efforts". Office arrangement or layout were also given considerable attention in order to avoid "wasted" time away from the desk.

In many ways, office work lends itself to rationalisation more than factory work. This can be attributed to the nature of the process itself: clerical operations are conducted almost entirely on paper, and paper is easier than industrial products to move, rearrange, combine or recombine, and so forth; and much of the "raw material" of clerical work is numerical in form, which facilitates the structuring of the process according to mathematical rules, particularly standardisation, verification and control. However, in spite of efforts to separate conception from execution, the use of the brain is never completely eliminated—any more than it is entirely done away with in any form of manual work. The mental processes are rendered repetitious and routine, and are reduced to a small part of the work process as the speed and dexterity with which manual operations are performed dominate the content of the job. Gradually, the traditional distinctions between the office as the site of mental labour and the factory shop-floor as the site of manual labour became blurred.

With the trend towards specialisation and the development of mechanisation, there grew the tendency to arrange or concentrate machines on a functional basis. Typing pools were established and extensively used. Organising work in this way was said to contribute to a more efficient use of machines and better control over the work process. This concentration of machines according to their functions, together with the workers who operated them, entrenched job specialisation as a guiding principle in office organisation.

The fragmentation and rationalisation of office work based on the principles of scientific management still exist. Paradoxically, Taylor's scientific management on the factory shop-floor initially enriched the jobs of the staff in offices. Today, however, many office workers are essentially semi-skilled machine operators, and pooling arrangements persist.

The mechanisation of office work

The early "scientific" office managers, like Taylor, were primarily concerned with rationalising existing procedures rather than with the mechanisation of the office. Although the typewriter was used widely and adding, dictating and ledger-posting mechanical devices had already been introduced, they took the existing level of technological development as given. As in the factory, solutions to problems of organisational size and complexity were first found in the technical division of labour, specifically through scientific management, and then through technology, specifically through mechanisation.

The first office machines were designed to perform single functions. Typewriters eliminated the tedious work of recording data by hand. Adding machines enabled the worker to perform rapidly most of the simple calculations required in clerical work. The use of these simple machines, however, did not entail radical changes in job content and skill requirements. Rather, they replaced a great deal of laborious manual effort in copying and checking data, and routine arithmetical calculations. The skills required in this work had been mainly acquired through practice, and a good general education, a knowledge of office routines and some understanding of the business continued to be the desirable qualifications of the clerical worker, whether his work was done by manual or by mechanical means.

After the First World War, the second stage of mechanisation began with the invention of machines which combined several functions. These ranged from the still relatively simple adding machine, which computes and records, to more complex book-keeping machines, which print invoices as they perform calculations and post the data on a ledger card. Such multi-function machines reduced clerical skill requirements; training in accounting, for example, was no longer necessary for book-keeping clerks. These machines also laid the foundation for greater office specialisation.

The introduction of punched-card techniques and the application of electronic computers to data processing characterised the next stage of mechanisation. It also marked the first phase of the computer's modern history and the emergence of the kind of data-entry work which is the focus of this book.

The type of mechanical action underlying punched-card systems of data processing profoundly changed the nature of clerical work. As noted earlier, the specialisation of functions and the rationalisation of office work had already begun to develop prior to this stage of mechanisation, owing to the increase in the volume of office work. Once the volume of data processed by offices became sufficiently great, the tendency towards job specialisation was intensified and the employment of full-time staff to punch cards was justified. An increasing number of employees were generally assigned exclusively to operate special-purpose machines, such as the keypunch, as their sole function. Data entry became an occupation as well as a task.

Punched-card data processing introduced into the office the type of mechanisation analogous to that found in assembly lines in factories. Tasks formerly done by hand could now be processed through the use of special-purpose machines upon which this system of data processing was based. There was a one-to-one relationship between the operator and the machine.

As previously mentioned, the typewriter was invented in the early stage of office mechanisation. The typewriter facilitated the entrance of women into the clerical labour force and changed office procedures. Its widespread use and the increasing tendency towards job specialisation made possible new organisational models, such as the typing or secretarial pool. According to Shepard, "the secretarial pool, where female clerks type on a full-time basis, is an excellent example of the employment of a low-level technological device to create a number of specialised, machine-operating jobs".[11] Manual dexterity became an important skill requirement for the operators of these machines.

The typewriter went through a series of technical improvements. In 1964, International Business Machines introduced the Magnetic Tape Selectric Typewriter, commonly referred to as the "MT/ST". The MT/ST made it possible not only to record a document and play it back, but also to edit or correct the text by rerunning it and making the necessary amendments. The MT/ST is generally considered the precursor of today's word-processing equipment. With advances in microelectronics, more sophisticated machines have appeared on the market.

MODERN DATA ENTRY: EQUIPMENT AND TASKS

The introduction of electronic computers facilitated the processing and storage of vast amounts of data. However, the electronic computer is still linked with the punched-card mode of data processing. Rather than completely superseding or eliminating the punched-card system, electronic data processing (EDP) technology makes use of special-purpose machines for input and output functions. For this reason, not all employees in an EDP unit are affected by automation. Employees who operate machines auxiliary or peripheral to the computer remain semi-skilled operators in a mechanised environment. Of course, the punched card may have been replaced by direct entry to tapes or discs, but the task of data preparation remains the same.

A similar process of technological advancement also altered the hardware used by typists; but there, too, workers have been left with essentially the same task. Just as full-time keypunchers appeared as a result of the increase in the volume of data to be processed, the widespread use of electronic computers and the intensification of office rationalisation, similar events led to the proliferation of full-time typists.

Keypunching

The machine originally used is commonly referred to as the "keypunch". It is used to punch holes in cards from a keyboard that resembles that of a standard typewriter.

The operator reads the source document and, by depressing the proper key, converts the information into punches or holes in the card. By pressing other keys, the operator can also skip or space over predetermined card columns or fields, duplicate into the next card information from the preceding card, and position or eject cards. An experienced operator can produce some 8,000–10,000 key-strokes an hour.

In some cases, keypunch operators are also responsible for verification. In this case, a card verifier is used which is similar to the keypunch but only senses punched data. The operator reads the same source document used for the original keypunching and depresses the same keys on the keyboard. A difference in what has been punched and what the operator enters causes the machine to stop. A notch will then be cut in the top of the card for visual reference later in the correction stage. Verification requires 100 per cent repetition of the original keying.

EDP changed the nature of clerical work, particularly for those workers who became full-time operators of special-purpose office machines. In the American civil service, keypunch operators have been classified not as "office workers" but as "machine operators".[12] A United States Department of Labor publication indicates that the keypunch operator should have a "preference for organised and routine activities to transfer data on to punch cards", that she should be "able to perform repetitive duties of operating a keypunch machine", and that she should have the "ability to follow instructions and set procedures to transfer data on to punch cards".[13]

Word processing

In spite of its common use, there is no agreed definition of the term "word processing". Manufacturers tend to define word processing in terms of the facilities their equipment provides, and users in terms of their requirements or the characteristics of installed systems.[14]

Broad definitions of word processing can cover all manipulation, dissemination and storage of textual information, i.e. everything from typing through copying to filing.

A more restricted definition of word processing, which we shall use in this study, is "the application of computer-based techniques to facilitate the tasks associated with the preparation and production of typed text".[15] Word processing is thus interpreted as a step towards the automation of typing functions.

There is an extensive range of word processors available. In many cases, the equipment is referred to as a visual display unit (VDU) or visual display terminal (VDT).[16] Most such equipment has the following main components:

(a) an electronic keyboard (similar to a conventional typewriter keyboard but with extra keys to give instructions to the machine);

(b) a visual display screen (for displaying the text typed or retrieved from memory);

(c) a central processing unit (a computer or microprocessor pro- grammed to interpret the instructions fed into it by the operator and to control the output. It usually also incorporates an internal memory store to hold input information);

(d) a storage unit (usually discs for keeping standard texts and docu- ments to be printed); and

(e) a printer.

Word-processing equipment is not merely a sophisticated typewriter. It has functions conventional typewriters do not have and often performs similar tasks in a different way. These capabilities are designed to help the word-processing operator to speed up the initial text keying and minimise layout problems, to allow modifications to the text recorded or stored in the computer's memory, to facilitate the use of text already stored to create a new document, and to improve the quality of the printed text.[17] Most word-processing equipment has the following distinctive capabilities:

(1) *Input promoting and verification.* Since many documents have fixed passages (e.g. standard paragraphs in letters or parts of reports), these can be automatically supplied by the computer. This means that the operator need respond only to specific queries. Prompting is usually in the form of "menu" displays which ask the operator whether she wants to edit an old document or print an existing one.

(2) *Text editing.* Once the text is keyed and stored, it can easily be amended. Words, lines, paragraphs or even pages can be deleted, altered, transposed or corrected easily and rapidly. Text can be reorganised in a new format; pages can be automatically renumbered to accommodate changes in text, and so on.

(3) *Error correction.* Word processing allows for corrections to be made by retyping only the offending words or passages. Since the correction is made to the "copy" in the machine's memory, the final printed version is perfect.

(4) *Text storage and retrieval.* Standard letters, paragraphs, parts of reports, etc., can be stored and easily reproduced. Some word-processing units also provide an extremely efficient, high-density, random-access filing system allowing large quantities of data to be stored in a remarkably small space.

Essentially, these capabilities mean that the word-processing operator can type faster, type less on each document and type for more of the working time available.[18] For example, she can type faster because the above-mentioned facilities provide faster input, faster correction (typist's errors) and faster editing (author's changes). She types less because the storage and retrieval capacities of the equipment enable her to re-use certain standard texts, and because she needs to retype only corrections or amendments. She can type for more of the time available because the separation of input and printing means the elimination of paper and carbon handling, and because less time is spent on changing margins, planning layouts and format, renumbering pages, and so on.

These capabilities indicate that there are a large number of possible applications. A few examples are cited below—

(1) *Form letters and similar documents.* The ideal use of word processing is, of course, where existing typing work involves a large amount of repetitive work, as in the case of form letters. A typist may call on to her screen a standard letter and fill in the blanks. The text surrounding the entries is then reorganised and printed, giving the impression of a tailor-made personalised letter.

(2) *Standard texts.* Another common application is the recombination of standard texts. When standard paragraphs are quoted, such as in insurance, they can be called on to the word processor from storage and put together to form a letter or document. Additional texts or changes can be typed in where desired. In some cases, a large number of letters are sent which consist of various recombinations of standard paragraphs, with the occasional variable text written in. Instead of writing all the paragraphs, the author has a list of all standard paragraphs with code numbers as identifiers. He then merely inserts the name of the person to whom the letter is addressed and adds the code numbers of the relevant paragraphs and any original text to be added. The typist simply keys the paragraph number as defined, together with any intermediate original text, and the system composes the whole letter to be printed.

Example 1[22]

ASSOCIATE CORRESPONDENCE SECRETARY

Reports to: word-processing supervisor or co-ordinator.
Basic functions: serves the company by using transcribing equipment, handwritten source material or abstracts of printed material, and prepares by recording on a text-editing typewriter the following:
—general correspondence;
—routine proposals;
—dictation requests for proof-reading and error correction on playback of final copy.
Responsibilities:
—may attend one or more text-editing typewriters. Plays back and merges material for repetitive letters;
—keyboards input and plays back final output;
—types a variety of assignments in the area of transcription, draft copy-typing, and composing, as required;
—types from wide variety of source documents;
—develops efficient work station management methods such as collating carbon copies or proof-reading while text editor is playing back final copy.
—performs related tasks as required by the supervisor.

Reprinted with permission of the Dartnell Corporation.

Example 2[23]

WORK FUNCTIONS IN A WORD-PROCESSING SYSTEM

Function	Other job titles used to mean same position	Responsibilities or tasks	Characteristics needed for the job
Correspondence (Persons who operate word-processing equipment/ have typing responsibilities)	*Correspondence secretary* Word-processing secretary Word-processing operator Word-processing specialist Word-processing co-ordinator Word processor Operators: Mag Card,[1] MC/ST,[2] MT/ST,[3] ATS[4] Typist: power typist; word-processing typist Transcription specialist Typing correspondence specialist Proof-reader Junior correspondence secretary Equipment operator Text editor operator Document specialist	Type fast Produce error-free copy Proof-read Correct errors Manage time Set work priorities Possibly take dictation Machine transcribe Do high volume of work Do quality work Collate and possibly distribute work	Positive attitude Like to type Analytical/abstract ability Machine oriented Machanical aptitude Technical ability Ability to understand new equipment/ terminology Enjoy working with equipment Able to accept challenges/change Conscientious to detail Self-directive, a "doer" Loyalty Ability to handle pressure Confidentiality Accept criticism, flexible Work with interruptions Like team-work/ co-operative

[1] Magnetic card.   [2] Magnetic Card Selectric Typewriter.   [3] Magnetic Tape Selectric Typewriter.
[4] Administrative Terminal System.

---

(3) *Report production.* Another suitable use of word processing is the production of bulky reports. When amendments are made to long typewritten drafts, the process of retyping is time-consuming and often compromises have to be made to expedite the completion of the report. This is especially true if changes are made in the first part of the report and the typist has to retype the whole report just to tidy it up. Word processors are particularly suited to such tasks. If corrections are made by the author to the original draft, the whole report does not need to be retyped. Depending on storage capacity, the report can be kept on disc until it is amended and/or printed in "top copy" form.

(4) *Specialised applications.* Some specialised uses, based on those described above, are found in mail order houses and the like. These include, for example, the sending of standard letters to prospective clients according to a classification index. Thus, if a mailing house

Example 3[24]

QUALITIES REQUIRED IN A WORD-PROCESSING OPERATOR

Job specification:

It is essential that the new recruit is aware that the job will be, in many offices, 99 per cent straight typing. It is highly unlikely that an expensive system will be left idle for hours on end while the operator does filing, photocopying or answers the telephone. In most offices the word-processing machine is used as a work-horse to deal with either the heavily edited work or the repetitive systems, and is often shared by several departments and is therefore in constant demand. It is important, therefore, that the word-processing operator has no illusions about the volume of typing.

There is, however, a more attractive side to the job, especially if the system is totally new. Setting up new systems, logging and filing are very demanding and most operators enjoy this creative side of the job. As the operator is often best aware of the capabilities of the machine, he/she is frequently best able to suggest more efficient methods of achieving the same result, replacing many an outdated procedure, in other words by developing new ways of doing work. With technology changing constantly, it is wise for the operator to keep abreast of the times, especially in the consumables area which is becoming highly competitive.

To sum up, the job may at first appear to be just slog typing, but this is by no means the case given the right encouragement and scope.

Remember: THE MACHINE IS ONLY AS GOOD AS THE OPERATOR

Operator requirements:

An accurate typist is essential, as it is a fallacy that the initial editing facility aids the typist. Experience shows that an inaccurate typist often becomes lazier when working a word-processing machine, to the extent that any time saved by the machine in producing a document is lost by the extensive revisions that have to be carried out after the work is checked.

A logical mind and an interest in machinery is an essential requirement. Also, the nature of all word-processing machines demands a high degree of concentration, especially if there is more than one system in a room.

To be totally effective in the job, the girl must be organised and dedicated. To employ an operator with a sense of challenge is always a good basis for setting up a new system.

wants to send different letters to male and female prospective clients, the system may be instructed to address one particular standard letter to males and another to females. Other classification criteria may be used, as long as they are coded in the original list.

However, the extent to which the above possible applications are actually used depends on the type of VDU task. In general, VDU tasks fall into three main categories: data entry, dialogue-type tasks and data inquiry.[19]

When the VDU is used mainly for data entry, the principal activities which are performed by the operator involve (*a*) reading a source document of one kind or another, and (*b*) entering this information into the computer through the keyboard. Operators engaged in data-entry

19

tasks are usually highly skilled in typing, so the speed with which the data are entered is relatively high. The present study is concerned with this type of VDU task.

In dialogue-type tasks, the activity is characterised by the flow of information from a document or person as a data source to the computer store and vice versa. Operators performing this type of VDU task do not usually need the same level of typing skill as data-entry personnel.

The principal activity in data inquiry VDU tasks is requesting information from the computer store. Like operators engaged in dialogue-type tasks, operators rarely command the same typing skill as data-entry operators.

The introduction of word-processing systems is radically changing the traditional office roles of secretaries and typists. Some of these changes will be discussed in the following chapters. Whether the changes are experienced as satisfactory or otherwise depends on a host of factors, such as the personal attributes and experiences of the workers involved, the organisational structure, and the design and content of jobs.

Exactly how secretaries and typists use word processing depends on the equipment, the word-load (i.e. the number of words that can be stored) and the configuration of the word-processing system.

Although there are many possible ways of organising word-processing systems, one of the most common ones seems to split the secretarial functions into two main jobs: typing and administration. As a management guide to word processing states: "Two separate functions and two separate groups of people to perform them: that is the essential 'specialisation' of the WP [Word Processing] approach".[20] This means the centralisation of all typing or data entry into a word-processing centre or unit. All other non-typing tasks, such as filing, answering telephones, scheduling appointments, ordering supplies, handling the mail, keeping records and charts, and so forth, are taken over by an administrative support centre. Although titles vary, workers in a word-processing centre are often called "word-processing operators" or "correspondence secretaries", while those in the administrative support centre are often called "administrative secretaries" or "administrative support secretaries".

Since the focus of this study is on full-time data-entry workers— word-processing operators or correspondence secretaries—in word-processing centres, it is important to see how work is typically organised in such centres.

The above-mentioned management guide gives an example: when work arrives (handwritten copy, typed manuscripts, dictation tapes, etc.), it is given a number and recorded in a log book. Typically, the supervisor (or co-ordinator, manager or administrator—titles vary) reviews the job to be done, sometimes with specific instructions from the "client", "originator" or "author", and determines how and by whom it will be done. The supervisor then attaches a job ticket and gives it to the word-processing operator for typing. Once the operator finishes typing the document, she gives it to the proof-reader or supervisor for checking. If there are corrections to be made, the job goes back to the operator. Otherwise it is sent to the author for review and signature, and the job ticket is completed and filed.[21]

There are many different job descriptions for word-processing operators. Some seek to emphasise job characteristics, such as the high level of skill required by complex company procedures, formats and machine operation. Others emphasise straightforward typing speed and accuracy. The examples given below of job descriptions illustrate differences in task requirements or at least in the way they are described in different word-processing situations.

PRESENT AND FUTURE EXTENT OF DATA-ENTRY JOBS

It is difficult to determine precisely the extent and future trend of data-entry jobs. Indeed, data-entry jobs and office work are found in all industries. Since we are dealing with a particular kind of work which is not confined to certain industries, statistical information is difficult to obtain.

Data-entry jobs are usually classified under either clerical or computer occupations. However, even within these occupational classifications, the large number and ambiguity of job titles make it difficult to identify which jobs involve full-time data entry. For example, in a survey of 17 operating companies within the Bell Telephone System alone in the United States, the Communication Workers of America found that in the clerical field there were 371 different job titles related to 84 pay grades. Not one of the 371 job titles was common to all companies, and on average each company shared only one or two titles with another.[25] Similarly, in a survey of computer workers, 170 respondents reported 71 distinct job titles.[26] Unfortunately, job titles do not necessarily reflect actual job content.

In spite of these difficulties, some estimates of the number of keypunch operators are available. On the basis of replies to the United States 1970 census, it was estimated that there were approximately 123,000 keypunch operators in 1965, increasing to 287,000 in 1970.[27]

It was only in 1972 that the United States Bureau of Labor Statistics (BLS) officially acknowledged the growth of EDP and the division of labour by including the occupations of computer operator, computer programmer and systems analyst in its national wages survey.[28] The BLS had for some years included keypunch operators as a category of office workers together with messengers, typists, tabulating machine operators, and the like. However, it acknowledged the number of workers in EDP occupations by including keypunch operators in its 1972-73 wages survey, covering 14,000 organisations employing nearly 10 million workers. The survey found 119,000 keypunch operators as compared with 51,000 computer operators, 42,000 computer programmers and 32,000 systems analysts. The insurance and banking industries were found to be the main employers of EDP workers. Unfortunately, the survey excluded the government sector.

The more comprehensive 1978 American labour force statistics cite 283,000 keypunch operators, 284,000 computer and auxiliary operators, 230,000 computer programmers and 160,000 systems analysts.[29] In 1983, BLS stated that there were 319,000 "data-entry operators" in 1979 and 320,000 in 1982, and projected a moderate decrease to 286,000 by 1995.[30] However, it is not clear if "data-entry operator" is merely a new label for "keypunchers". The same study also included typists, bank tellers, clerical supervisors, general office clerks and secretaries among the 40 occupations with largest job growth, and EDP peripheral equipment operators, medical insurance clerks and credit clerks in banking and insurance among the 20 fastest-growing occupations.[31]

In sum, the overall lack of statistical data, the ambiguity of job titles, the inconsistency of occupational classifications and the difficulty in isolating data-entry jobs, particularly word-processing jobs, from broad occupational categories mean that there is a need to consider indirect indicators of the present and future extent of data-entry jobs.

One indicator is the rapid growth of the market for word processors. In the United States, word processor sales of over $3,000 million were expected in 1984, with the potential to reach $4,200 million by 1987.[32] Moreover, a report on the American situation notes that the number of word-processing and data-processing terminals will triple from 7 million to 22 million in the next five years and that by 1985 some 27 million electronic office devices will be installed.[33] By 1985, according to an analysis of 1,400 American manufacturing companies, 100 per cent of secretaries will have work stations.[34]

In the United Kingdom, a survey of 255 companies found that 86 per cent were using electronic typewriters, 79 per cent word processors and 78 per cent micro-computers.[35] Moreover, a survey of local authorities found that 60 per cent were using word processors.[36]

The range of models available is another indication of the growth of the market. There are now over 100 different models of word processor on the market, excluding software packages (sets of programmes) which enable micro-computers to have the extra facility of word processing.[37] In the United Kingdom, the 94 per cent increase between 1981 and 1982 in sales of word-processing software packages is evidence that many micro-computers at least have the capability of word processing.[38]

The above-mentioned information concerning the growth of the market for word processors provides an indication of the likely present and future extent of data-entry work. However, it is difficult to determine the extent to which these word processors are being used for full-time data-entry jobs.

Word-processing terminals have not completely superseded traditional data-entry equipment, such as the keypunch. In spite of the predicted demise of such equipment, it continues to be used for data-entry in many situations.[39] There is still a large installed base of keypunch devices, and it is likely that they will retain a viable share of the market in spite of a predicted 8.2 per cent sales decline over the period 1980-85.[40]

Notes

[1] Jon M. Shepard: *Automation and alienation: A study of office and factory workers* (Cambridge, Massachusetts, and London, MIT Press, 1971), pp. 41–42.

[2] See, for example, Harry Braverman: *Labor and monopoly capital: The degradation of work in the twentieth century* (New York and London, Monthly Review Press, 1974), p. 295; Evelyn Nakano Glenn and Roslyn L. Feldberg: "Degraded and deskilled: The proletarianisation of clerical work", in *Social Problems* (New York), Oct. 1977, pp. 52–64 and Enid Mumford and Olive Banks: *The computer and the clerk* (London, Routledge and Kegan Paul, 1967), p. 19.

[3] Max Weber: "Bureaucracy", in H. Gerth and C. Wright Mills: *From Max Weber: Essays in sociology* (London, Oxford University Press, 1946), cited in Jay M. Shafritz and Philip H. Whitbeck (eds.): *Classics of organisation theory* (Oak Park, Illinois, Moore Publishing Co., 1978), pp. 37–42.

[4] Grace Coyle: "Women in the clerical occupations", in *The Annals, American Academy of Political and Social Sciences*, No. 143 (1929), pp. 180–187, cited in Evelyn Nakano Glenn and Roslyn L. Feldberg: "Clerical work: The female occupation", in *Working Woman* (New York, n.d.), p. 320.

[5] Frederick Winslow Taylor: *The principles of scientific management* (New York and London, Harper, 1919).

[6] idem: *Shop management* (New York and London, Harper, 1919), pp. 98–99.

[7] idem: *The principles of scientific management*, op. cit., p. 39.

[8] William H. Leffingwell: *Scientific office management* (New York, 1917), cited in Braverman, op. cit., p. 307.

[9] Charles Babbage: *On the economy of machinery and manufactures* (London, 1835; reprinted ed., New York, Kelley, 1963).

[10] Lee Galloway: *Office management: Its principles and practice* (New York, 1918), cited in Braverman, op. cit., pp. 306–307.

[11] Shepard, op. cit., p. 44.

[12] Ida Russakoff Hoos: "The impact of office automation on workers", in *International Labour Review*, Oct. 1960, p. 373.

[13] United States Department of Labor, Bureau of Employment Security: *Occupations in electronic computing systems* (Washington, DC, United States Government Printing Office, 1965), pp. 30 and 42, cited in Shepard, op. cit., p. 53.

[14] Infotech Ltd.: *Office automation: Analysis*, Infotech State of the Art Report, Series 8, No. 3 (Maidenhead, United Kingdom, 1980), p. 77.

[15] H-P. G. Kelly: "The use and usefulness of word processing", in Infotech Ltd.: *Office automation: Invited papers*, Infotech State of the Art Report, Series 8, No. 3 (Maidenhead, United Kingdom, 1980), p. 99.

[16] In this book, for the sake of consistency, we use the term "visual display unit (VDU)" throughout.

[17] S. G. Price: *Introducing the electronic office* (Manchester, National Computing Centre Ltd., 1979), p. 35.

[18] C. W. Blakely: "Word processing in the typing pool and the secretarial environment", in Infotech Ltd.: *Office automation: Invited papers*, op. cit., pp. 23–24.

[19] Not all VDU tasks can be exactly classified into one of these categories. Moreover, the dividing lines between them are not very precise and one can easily add other categories.

[20] Walter A. Kleinschrod: *Management's guide to word processing* (Chicago, Dartnell Corporation, 1977), p. 4.

[21] ibid., p. 42.

[22] ibid., p. 121.

[23] Marly Bergerud and Jean Gonzalez: *Word processing: Concepts and careers* (New York & Chichester, John Wiley, 1978), p. 168.

[24] Christine Davis: "Word processing staff and the rate for the job", in Online Conferences Ltd.: *Word processing: Selection, implementation and uses* (Uxbridge, United Kingdom, 1979), pp. 127–128.

[25] Phyllis M. Palmer and Sharon Grant: *The status of clerical workers: A summary analysis of research findings and trends* (1979; mimeographed).

[26] Donileen R. Loseke and John A. Sonquist: "The computer worker in the labor force: New occupations and old problems", in *Sociology of Work and Occupations* (Beverly Hills, California, and London), May 1979, p. 164.

[27] Author's calculations made from Teresa A. Sullivan and Daniel B. Cornfield: "Downgrading computer workers: Evidence from occupational and industrial redistribution", ibid., p. 194, table 2.

[28] James C. Taylor: *Fragmented office jobs and the computer* (Geneva, ILO, 1978; mimeographed internal working document; restricted), p. 2.

[29] United States Department of Labor, Bureau of Labor Statistics: *Occupational Outlook Handbook, 1978* (Washington, DC, 1978).

[30] George T. Silvestri et al.: "Occupational employment projections through 1995", in *Monthly Labor Review* (Washington, DC), Nov. 1983, p. 40, table 1.

[31] ibid., tables 2 and 3.

[32] Louise Kehoe: "US market becomes a battleground", in *Financial Times* (London), Special feature on the Desk Top Revolution, 16 Apr. 1984, p. xvi.

[33] Alan Cane: "Savings hard to identify", ibid., p. xx.

[34] ibid.

[35] *The Guardian* (London), 1 Sep. 1983.

[36] *Labour Research* (London), Nov. 1983, p. 276.

[37] R. Garner and M. Coffey, in *Computing Europe* (London), 4 Mar. 1982.

[38] *Labour Research*, op. cit., p. 276.

[39] "Demand for skilled operators exceeds supply", in *Computerworld*, 28 Apr. 1980.

[40] "Data-entry projected to retain market viability", in *Computerworld*, 22 Sep. 1980, p. 78.

DATA-ENTRY WORK: WORK ORGANISATION AND WORKING TIME

2

WORK ORGANISATION AND JOB CONTENT

Work organisation and job content are the main aspects of conditions of work which are affected by the introduction of computerisation, particularly by recent developments involving microprocessors. Specifically, computerisation is changing the worker's autonomy, responsibility and control over her work; the volume, intensity and pace of work; skills and careers; and communication and social support.

The following exposition and analysis tends to highlight problems often associated with the application of computer technology. This should not be construed as denying or minimising its positive outcomes or benefits, some of which are mentioned in the Introduction to this book. However, the emphasis has been put on problems in order to focus awareness and action where the needs are greatest. Awareness of negative effects may encourage choices in machines and in types of work organisation that explicitly take into account the effects of office technology on the conditions of work and quality of working life of data-entry workers. As various studies have shown, fragmentation of office work is a choice, not a technological imperative. Office technology is often viewed as a mixture of great potential benefits and great potential hazards. As too often before, its benefits tend to be over-sold and the question of cost to the worker evaded.

Autonomy, responsibility and control

One of the most striking characteristics of data-entry jobs is the lack of worker responsibility, autonomy and control on the job. Autonomy on the job refers to "the degree to which the job provides substantial freedom, independence and discretion to the individual in scheduling the work and in determining the procedures to be used in carrying it out".[1] It includes, for example, the amount of worker latitude in selection of work methods, work sequence, work pace and acceptance or rejection of the quality of incoming materials. Autonomy is an important job dimension in contributing to the workers' feeling of responsibility for outcomes on the job. To the extent that autonomy is high, the more work outcomes will be viewed by workers as depending substantially on their own efforts, initiative and decisions—rather than on the adequacy of instructions from the boss or on a manual of job procedures. Of course, to the extent that the job allows the worker autonomy and responsibility, the more likely she will be to perceive that she has control over her own work.

To what extent are these job characteristics found in data-entry work?

The standardisation and rationalisation that tend to accompany the application of computerised systems often take the form of further subdivision of work functions, the consolidation of similar or related tasks and activities, and the formalisation of the work process through emphasis on schedules, procedures and regulations.

As previously mentioned, one of the most common organising principles in word processing is the division of traditional secretarial work into two separate functions: typing and administration (non-typing). In many cases, word-processing centres are either former typing pools or have been established to centralise the typing function. For example, in a study of a bank in the United States, the word-processing centre was established "to replace typing work done by departmental secretaries throughout the bank with a centralised typing service".[2] It was divided into units based on the type of word-processing equipment used: a "Mag card" (magnetic card) unit, a Word plex unit and a Vydec unit, each with a supervisor. Under the supervisor were four specialist groups: machine or data-entry operators ("correspondence secretaries"), proof-readers ("quality assurance specialists"), and "input clerks" and "output clerks" who handled the interface tasks of classifying incoming work and preparing output documents respectively.[3] Of course, there may be variations in the division of labour. None the less, the secretarial function has been fragmented into discrete tasks or operations and subdivided among different groups of workers, with those performing the same operation concentrated in a particular area or "work station".

In such circumstances, data-entry workers have little or no discretion in scheduling or checking their work. The supervisor allocates and schedules work, and the proof-reader (or the supervisor) checks it. Partially owing to the greater interdependence among units or departments and greater dependence on hardware, certain tasks have to be carried out at specified times, in specified sequences, in prescribed forms and in prescribed ways.

Moreover, the extensive subdivision and simplification of the job, coupled with the concentration in a particular area of workers performing the same task, mean that most data-entry workers have little sense of the overall task to which they are contributing, or of how the system functions as a whole. This loss of "meaningfulness" makes any attempt to exercise responsibility and autonomy a difficult and frustrating experience.

A decrease in autonomy and responsibility is also reinforced by the introduction of work simplification, specialisation, and time and motion efficiency techniques long associated with factory work. In some cases, monitoring devices are incorporated into word processors. These devices not only measure key depressions and time spent on the machine but also issue instructions concerning how to do a specific job or signal disciplinary warnings if input speeds or time at the machine do not meet management targets. One can imagine a novice typist using this information to gauge her progress. "However, most systems that track productivity statistics do not make them available to the typist at all. Rather they report them to a supervisor, who can then use them for external performance evaluation".[4] Furthermore, "in some keypunching departments, each machine is wired to the supervisor board. By watching the lights on her board, the supervisor can tell immediately when any operator in the room stops punching".[5]

The simplification and standardisation of work also facilitate close supervision. Subdivided work with inflexible routines makes it easier for the supervisor to see to it that data-entry workers do their work accurately and meet their quotas on time. The job has been reduced to quantifiable elements, such as number of pages keyed, number of errors made, and so on. Thus, the nature of the task itself, combined with close supervision, restricts the workers' autonomy on the job and also increases their vulnerability.

The misapplication of word-processing technology has thus severely circumscribed workers' responsibility, autonomy and control on the job. The over-rationalisation of clerical procedures and processes has resulted in jobs which are repetitive and disjointed and offer little scope for personal initiative. These have often given rise to feelings of boredom, monotony and meaninglessness of work, loss of self-esteem and mental strain. It is, therefore, not surprising that full-time data entry is often said to resemble assembly-line work in manufacturing. Reduced to simple machine operators where the task of typing or encoding is the whole job, data-entry workers have little or no scope for experiencing responsibility, autonomy and control on the job.

Workload, work intensity and work pace

These job characteristics have become the focus of increasing attention in recent years. Because they require in-depth analysis and because they are especially closely related with symptoms of un-desirable work—stress and fatigue—they are considered separately in Chapter 4.

Skills and careers

One of the major effects of computerisation and the application of scientific management techniques to work content is the progressive elimination of opportunities for development and fuller use of skills and career advancement. In many cases, work methods have been altered in ways which render existing skills obsolete, devalue previous experience and reduce career prospects and occupational mobility.

In this section we examine the skill requirements of data-entry jobs, the characteristics of workers, the congruence between these two factors and their implications for career development.

Skill requirements

The skills required of data-entry workers can often be derived from job descriptions. Although these job descriptions may vary according to particular business operations, they often have some skill requirements in common. For example, as noted in Chapter 1, job descriptions for word-processing operators vary in the range of skills considered essential to job performance. However, a high level of typing skill (speed and accuracy) is the most important requirement. Some also emphasise proficiency in spelling and good understanding of punctuation rules. However, certain factors may mitigate against the worker's utilising or improving her knowledge of spelling or punctuation. In the division of labour in most word-processing units, tasks related to checking or editing text are allocated to the proof-reader, editor or supervisor. Pressure to maintain output also discourages the worker from any activity which may divert her from the keying task. She has a production quota to meet, and correcting spelling and punctuation mistakes will just slow her down. Moreover, the capabilities of the machine (such as its ability to correct mistakes) may reduce the gap between good and bad typists and thereby eliminate incentives to improve or widen one's skills.

For keypunching, the skill requirements focus on manual dexterity and keying. Skill in spelling and punctuation are irrelevant since the keypunching task consists of entering mostly numerical data on to cards, discs or tapes. Even the closely related task of verification merely entails re-keying or re-entering the same data. Moreover—

Data processing by machine is, in fact, as has often been stated, more akin to factory production work . . . since the attentiveness and mechanical skill of the machine operators are, on the whole, of greater importance than either their general educational background or business experience.[6]

To a great extent, the duration and content of training needed for users of these technologies is an indicator of the level and variety of skill requirements. Most of the training or retraining to acquire new skills to operate the equipment is provided on the job. Training can be provided by the manufacturer, the organisation or by self-taught (self-help) methods using programmed learning or training "diskettes" (i.e. floppy discs) provided by the manufacturers. Initial courses, however, are generally provided by the manufacturer or the supplier of the equipment. These courses tend to be quite short, often lasting not more than one week.[7] Their content usually covers the actual operation of the machine and the application of software. For example, in a study of data-entry workers in computing centres in Poland, it was noted that the most common kind of vocational training was on-the-job training during the first two weeks, where "the most important skill to be mastered is 'fingering' the keyboard . . .".[8]

Most workers report that it is easy to learn to operate the terminal, especially for data-entry tasks.[9] This is not surprising, since one of the criteria of a "good system" is that it "should be simple enough to use that the input operator, the typist, does not need extensive training".[10] In fact, ease of use is one of the advantages claimed by manufacturers.[11] Moreover, "the [word-processing] system is so simple to understand and to use—you'll begin to get your work back within *days* of installation".[12]

In some cases, additional training may be provided to learn the advanced applications or functions. However, this is often limited to supervisors or a few leading operators.

Similarly in the past, for using punched-card machinery, "the new skills did not present any great difficulty" and a brief on-the-job training proved sufficient regardless of the worker's background and previous work experience.[13] Today, this type of data-entry worker may work either using tapes or directly on-line as opposed to punched cards, "but these skills are not substantially different from the former ones . . .".[14]

The skill requirements of data-entry jobs are such that anyone can easily be trained to replace anyone else. This interchangeability and replaceability of data-entry workers is another reason why the distinction between office and factory work is said to be disappearing.

In designing these jobs, the assumption seems to be that an effective way to increase "skilfulness" or assure depth of skill in one area is to restrict the overall range of skills in other areas to the absolute minimum.[15]

Workers' characteristics

Thus far the skill requirements of data-entry jobs have been described. However, since a "good" job is a function of both the characteristics of workers and the characteristics of the work performed, the degree of congruence between them can affect substantially the impact of the job on worker satisfaction and productivity. It is, therefore, necessary to consider the characteristics—educational background, skills, preferences, attitudes, etc.—of data-entry workers.

Data-entry workers come from varied backgrounds. This hetero-geneity is increasing as the word processor is used in an increasing number of business operations. Most data-entry workers have at least a full secondary education, which indeed is often a prerequisite for initial employment. For example, in a survey of word-processing centres in 30 organisations in New York City, a high-school education was considered one of the "minimum qualifications" for entry-level word-processing positions.[16] For key-punching jobs, most employers also specify a high-school diploma.

Apart from their secondary education, many data-entry workers receive training in stenography or other special subjects from vocational or commercial institutions.

While it is difficult to separate data-entry workers from the broader category of clerical workers, it is likely that a certain proportion of data-entry workers have some college or university education. In the United States, for example, nearly one in four adult workers today has a university degree as compared to one in seven in 1970.[17] Between 1970 and 1983 the number of workers aged 25–64 with four years or more of college education increased by 11.4 million. Almost half of this rise was among the 25–34 age group with the 35–44 age group accounting for the rest. Moreover, while the proportion of male workers aged 25–64 with college degrees rose by more than two-thirds over the period from 1970 to 1983, that of women doubled. A 1976 demographic survey of educational attainment of 231 secretaries, stenographers and typists in a federal agency in Washington, DC, showed that the mean educational attainment was 13 years.[18] In 1979 it was estimated that 24.3 per cent of all clerical workers in the United States had at least some college education and that 7.0 per cent had four or more years.[19] Furthermore, because of the tight labour market, many workers are forced to be less selective about the job they are willing to take. It is not uncommon for a woman with a university degree to take a secretarial course or to rely on typing skills learned during secondary education in order to obtain a more available clerical job.

Just as data-entry workers vary in their educational attainment, they also differ in terms of their work experience. Some data-entry workers are recent graduates of secondary schools; some are typists in a typing pool who become word-processing operators in a word-processing pool; some are personal secretaries who become word-processor operators; and some are women who are re-entering the labour force after bearing children and attending to family responsibilities.

Data-entry workers also vary in their work attitudes and preferences. They differ, for example, in the degree to which work is a central interest; what the most important feature(s) of the work activity is; and the extent to which various aspects of the job are liked or disliked. For some workers, work or the job is merely a means to a pay packet, while for others it is an important part of life. Some prosper in simple routine work, whereas others prefer complex and challenging tasks. Some feel that work or the job should provide some economic security, if not necessarily psychological fulfilment.

For some, work provides an opportunity to form and maintain social relationships, while others see it as giving direction and purpose to their lives by structuring their time and getting them involved in some "useful" activity. And for some, particularly married women with children, it provides an identity separate from their family roles.

Data-entry workers are therefore typical of workers today in that they have increasingly different educational attainments, work attitudes, values and preferences. However, data-entry jobs often do not provide opportunities for them to use the various forms of knowledge and skill they have acquired in ways which suit their individual preferences.

Congruence between skills and workers' characteristics

A typical secretarial job consists of several tasks and activities as, for example, administrative work and filing, telephone and reception duties, as well as typing. It therefore provides more opportunities for the person to use a variety of skills and different levels of skill. The worker is likely to perceive that her skills are being adequately used and that she is being assisted to develop them and become increasingly competent. In such circumstances, there will probably be a good "fit" between the job requirements and the skills, knowledge and expectations of the worker, and this is likely to improve job satisfaction.

Moreover, since workers have different preferences or attitudes concerning various aspects or features of the job, a job which offers a variety or range of activities and tasks increases the likelihood that at least some of the individual preferences and expectations can be accommodated. For example, one person may have good interpersonal skills and may enjoy contacts with clients, while another may prefer keeping schedules of appointments, briefing her chief about clients, taking dictation and doing other tasks associated with being a "personal" assistant. Variety in the job can also minimise repetitiveness which often leads to boredom. The worker can fall back on alternative tasks and activities to relieve the monotony of certain tasks.

In contrast, the word-processing operator's job consists essentially of operating the word processor; in other words, typing. The extreme job simplification and specialisation mean that the worker's skills and knowledge are underutilised and that her opportunities for personal development are restricted. The skill requirements of the job—speed, accuracy and manual dexterity—relate mostly to mechanical skills. Most secretaries would consider this second type of job as a transition to increasingly machine-oriented work.

However, the extent to which the job is "deskilled" depends on the worker's previous experience. For example, the personal secretary whose job has been transformed into that of word-processing operator is likely to consider the change as deskilling, since it represents a considerable reduction in variety and discretion and an increase in task specialisation and devaluation of skills apart from typing. However, for the typist in a typing pool who becomes an operator in a word-processing pool, the change is not so dramatic as that of the personal secretary. In fact, it is argued that the technical capacity of the word processor reduces repetitive typing and thereby decreases job monotony; however, this is true only when the worker is subsequently given more varied tasks to do.

The introduction of word processing usually generates enthusiasm among clerical workers. They have positive expectations about learning new skills and having new jobs. There is usually an increase in job satisfaction. Unfortunately, this is often a temporary phenomenon. Once the data-entry worker has learned the capacities of the equipment, such as how to make amendments to text or to perform specific tasks to process certain documents, there is little more to learn. By allocating a large part of the work to the technology and leaving little to the discretion of the worker, the job has been reduced to such a level that, once the novelty of the technology has worn off, the dulling effects of routine activity take over.

The job becomes so devoid of skill variety that in some cases operator aptitude, rather than skill, is found to be critical in determining job satisfaction. For example, a company in the United Kingdom found that the best people to staff a word-processing centre were not the best typists but the people who most enjoyed working with machines.[20] Good copy-typists became frustrated with the word processor because it produced perfect copy independently of the quality of their skill; they felt that their jobs were deskilled and their skills downgraded.

In the 1960s, similar events occurred with respect to keypunching jobs. Employers who initially preferred to retrain their own staff for machine operation found that workers with little or no knowledge of commercial practice or office routines could be as quickly trained, and fitted in or adapted more easily to this type of work, than experienced personnel.

Changes are occurring between what people seek from a job and what the job provides. According to BLS, the growth in the number of adult workers with university degrees carries with it the possibility of an uncertain future for many graduates.[21] This is because the greatest increase in the number of jobs over the decade to come is projected for such occupations as janitors, sales clerks, secretaries and so forth. Thus, there is potentially a growing mismatch between actual educational levels and those required for occupations with the greatest anticipated growth. In a recent survey of London firms (where there is a secretarial shortage), personnel managers cited increased demands for challenging and interesting work as the main reason for their difficulties in recruiting and retraining secretaries.[22] The widening gap between workers' characteristics and the realities of the workplace implies that many workers in the future are likely to be underemployed and dissatisfied.

Career development

The discrepancy between deskilled jobs and rising educational attainment might be more easily accepted if workers could look forward to career progression after a period of routine work. Unfortunately, full-time data-entry jobs are often "dead-end" jobs where there is little or no chance of advancement.[23]

In most word-processing centres, a two-track career ladder is typical. One career ladder exists for administrative support secretaries and another for word-processing operators or correspondence secretaries. This system means that there are two hierarchies, each made up of jobs graded by level, representing career steps. A person who starts on the career ladder of word-processing operator may move up the ranks as she gains experience, but she is rarely allowed to cross over on to a different ladder. For example, she can move from data-entry operator I to data-entry operator II, but she cannot move to administrative secretary II. Although job titles may vary, a typical career ladder for word-processing operators consists of the following steps:

—associate or junior word-processing operator (or associate or junior correspondence secretary or data-entry operator I);

—word-processing operator (or correspondence secretary or data-entry operator II);

—senior or leading word-processing operator (or senior or leading correspondence secretary or data-entry operator III);

—data-entry supervisor (or correspondence centre supervisor).

Associate or junior word-processing operator is the entry-level step. However, the qualifications and activities for word-processing operator (data-entry operator II) and senior or leading word-processing operator (data-entry operator III) are often essentially the same, except that the latter requires greater proficiency in typing, particularly of more complex documents, and a more thorough knowledge of company standards and procedures; she also gives, instead of assists in, equipment demonstrations. The difference lies, therefore, in degree of proficiency in performing specific tasks rather than any actual increase in job content. This seems to illustrate the underlying assumption in the design of data-entry jobs, as previously mentioned: to increase "skilfulness" or depth of skill in one or two areas by restricting the overall range of skills.

The most obvious career opportunity for word-processing operators is promotion to word-processing supervisor. Supervisors are considered as first-level management. However, the position often does not lead to promotion to higher grades. Since a supervisor has essentially the same skills as the operators she supervises, she is also handicapped by the lack of skill requirements for promotion to senior positions, particularly those outside the word-processing hierarchy. Moreover, even this position may be eliminated eventually as equipment flexibility and capacity increase. Indeed, various supervisory levels can be eliminated by using machines which are capable of measuring the output and error rate of each employee. Some operators may reach supervisory positions rapidly and are then blocked as the job progression scale is closed to them. Many, however, will remain in the same grade or position for the rest of their working lives.

Several authors have observed that mechanisation and computerisation promote a levelling of the office structure to one with a large number of lower-grade jobs and few supervisory positions.[24] As a consequence of this truncated occupational structure, workers are likely to perceive that there is no opportunity for upward mobility for them in the hierarchy. It is thus understandable for people working in an occupational hierarchy with few possibilities for advancement to feel that promotions are achieved on grounds other than merit or ability.

In many ways, word-processing operator jobs move the worker out of the secretarial hierarchy which at least offered more, even if still limited, career opportunities. The work specialisation within word processing makes it difficult for an operator to acquire the skills and qualifications necessary for improving her occupational mobility and career prospects. The nature of the job prevents the worker from demonstrating her readiness for more responsible, varied and remunerative work. Moreover, even if an operator or secretary could easily learn the extra skills required, many company promotion regulations often specify that formal qualifications are needed.

The same career problems were experienced earlier by clerical employees when EDP was introduced in the 1960s. At that time, programming positions were considered to be part of management and it was said that many keypunchers could aspire to these positions. However, these workers did not qualify for the new positions since experience in coding, keypunching or checking was not so important as were certain analytical skills and educational background. Therefore, for the majority of clerical employees, programming jobs were outside the area of reasonable expectations.

After a relatively short time, many data-entry workers extinguish their hopes for advancement.[25] This limitation of aspiration, however, may not lead them to leave the firm; instead it leads them to discredit the idea of promotion by declaring that it is irrelevant and that they have no wish to be supervisors. As soon as they lose all hope of advancement, they tend to lose interest in everything not directly connected with their daily routine. The majority adopt the attitude: "I do my work and don't bother about the rest." The only claim they make on the organisation in exchange for their service is the right not to perform any other services.

In some cases, this lack of career opportunities can be hidden by the variety and ambiguity of job titles. As some studies have shown, job titles are not accurate indicators of job complexity and responsibility. In some cases, "new career paths may be more apparent than real".[26]

It is apparent that, for these workers, training is necessary for more senior positions, preferably outside the word-processing hierarchy. Access to training, however, can pose problems. For example, a survey of 53 organisations in London showed that firms rejected the concept of offices as "colleges for further education":[27] 30 per cent offered no training for secretaries or typists, while 20 per cent provided training which would help secretaries to perform more effectively in their present job, rather than giving them the chance of promotion. Some firms were more likely to pay for evening classes than to arrange training during working hours. The general view of means towards gaining promotion was that "it is up to the secretaries to make their own opportunities by *(a)* becoming involved, *(b)* gaining qualifications and *(c)* remembering they have to compete with others who may already have a degree or professional qualification".[28]

Consequently, for most of these workers, the "main avenues for mobility . . . are either horizontal or downward".[29] This was recognised as early as 1956 by the American Management Association, which stated in a special report to help employers to set up data-processing operations—

To be honest—we don't want people to take data-processing jobs as stepping-stones to other jobs. We want permanent employees capable of doing good work and satisfied to stay and do it. To promise rapid advancement is to falsify the facts. The only rapid advancement for the bulk of non-supervisory data-processing staff is *out of data processing!*[30]

In addition to a dearth of career opportunities, data-entry workers also lack job security. Just as a blue-collar assembly-line worker can be easily replaced, the data-entry worker in a highly rationalised job finds that she has a precarious hold on her position. Many data-entry workers are acutely aware that they are expendable.

Social support and communication

Definitions of social support vary, but the core idea is the communication of positive feelings—liking, trust and respect—by other significant people in one's life. Specifically—

. . . people may be said to have social support if they have a relationship with one or more other persons which is characterised by relatively frequent interactions, strong and positive feelings, and especially perceived ability and willingness to lend emotional and/or instrumental assistance in times of need.[31]

Existing empirical evidence suggests that supportive relationships satisfy important affiliative needs, and develop, enhance and confirm a person's sense of identity and self-esteem. Such relationships also facilitate problem-solving and the internalisation of and commitment to organisational goals. An important component of social support is communication among workers.

Computerisation and its accompanying organisational changes have transformed social relationships in the office. The excessive fragmentation and specialisation of work, the formation or entrenchment of pooling arrangements, and the standardisation of jobs, transactions and even of personal interactions have led to impersonal and apathetic relationships.

The data-entry task itself does not require interaction among workers. The job has been simplified and standardised so that the worker spends her time "interacting" with the terminal: that is, keying the text. Particularly within word-processing pools, there is no need for inter-dependence among workers, since everyone is doing the same thing. Work simplification has also led to high performance standards which leave little time for the worker to engage in conversations or face-to-face contacts with fellow-workers, except during rest breaks. Even during these breaks, the demands of the task sometimes leave the worker so mentally exhausted that she may prefer to be alone to "unwind". Of course, monitoring techniques also discourage interaction with fellow-workers.

Earlier studies have shown that, when the pressures towards productivity are very strong and the organisation of work is such that there is little interdependence between workers, the amount of social interaction will be low and solid supportive relationships will be rare.[32]

Moreover, as previously mentioned, highly fragmented work and the concentration in the same area of workers performing the same task prevent the worker from understanding the total work process. In addition to limiting the workers' potential scope for responsibility and autonomy, this situation makes it difficult for them to know what others in different units are doing, to share experiences and to provide mutual support. In some cases, this fragmentation is exacerbated by physical separation within the same building, in a separate building or in another geographical area. Geographical separation is gradually being facilitated by developments in telecommunications networks, distributed data processing and electronic mail. Nevertheless, workers usually resent the isolation which results. The possibilities for remote site working, particularly home work, may aggravate this isolation, as opportunities for face-to-face contact and companionship are eliminated.[33]

Even within the office, physical layout—particularly "open-plan" or "open" office [34]—may discourage significant social inter-action. "Line-of-sight geography", one of the characteristics of the open-plan office, allows visual observation of various work centres from a distant site, usually from the supervisor's location. This awareness of being under constant scrutiny prevents the workers from freely talking to each other, even during rest breaks. Moreover, some employees indicate that it is impossible in an open-plan office to engage in private conversation either with fellow-workers or with supervisors.[35]

In some open-plan offices, the modular work station configuration tends to intensify the worker's feeling of isolation. For example, a VDU operator explains the practice in a newspaper company as follows:

I work at a terminal all day. When the union pushed the newspaper company where I work, they improved the colours and lighting and all that for the full-time operators. Now they have a new set-up called "the open office". There are dark blue panels 6 feet high around all the operators. In many cases, we don't see another person all day except for a ten-minute break and lunchtime. All we see is the walls around us and the supervisor. The isolation is terrible.[36]

Moreover, certain practices (such as the posting of daily performance, incentive systems and exhortations) which encourage competition among workers may undermine group cohesiveness and the limited opportunities for social support. Even group incentive systems may lead to the expulsion or ostracism of members who do not meet performance standards. In these cases, workers often complain that they are treated "like children" or "like machines".

It is significant to note that, in most word-processing units, close supervision and the standardisation of work create conflicting pressures.[37] On the one hand, workers are tempted to relieve or minimise the problems and tensions at work through co-operation and solidarity. On the other hand, they feel vulnerable and thus their desire for personal relationships is decreased. Frequently, after several years of service, data-entry workers become reserved and suspicious towards colleagues, shy away from friendship and avoid social interaction with colleagues outside work.

The fragmentation of responsibility, together with the rigidity of bureaucratic organisations, means that contact with management may be limited and filtered through layers of supervisors. Although the supervisor is considered first-level management, owing to office rationalisation she is not part of the staff who "conceptualise" and "plan" the work, but rather part of the workers who are expected to carry it out. It is commonly said that the supervisor has two jobs: she must be concerned with her subordinates, and she must see that the work gets done. Accurate though the first part of the statement may be, the second is too simple. Supervisors do not produce the work by themselves. Instead, they structure the situation so that others can do their job more effectively.

In many cases, just as the factory foreman is the "man in the middle", the supervisor is the buffer between management and the workers. Being in the middle or boundary position means that the supervisor is likely to be caught between the demands of management and of those under her. Inasmuch as she is evaluated on the quantity and quality of output of her unit, she is likely to transfer the pressure under which she is working to the operators in her unit. In such circumstances, some supervisors may be tempted to resort to authority and sanctions to ensure that quality and quantity production standards are met. Recourse to such formal controls may lead to a climate of apathy, intimidation, frustration and low morale, and to "work-to-rule" behaviour. These, in turn, may result in low productivity, increased error rates, absenteeism, and so on. Of course, once this happens, even more formal controls become necessary and the vicious circle continues. Reliance on authority and sanctions can result in conformity and acquiescence, but not in enthusiastic co-operation.

Related to—or constituting a part of—social support is the process of communication, including feedback. There are many sources of feedback: the hardware, the proof-reader, the supervisor and/or the author.

The word-processing terminal provides the operator with auditory feedback apart from the different "cues" and "prompts". However, this type of feedback is very limited and concerns only the immediate task at hand. It relates purely to direct worker-machine interaction in its narrowest sense without giving the operator any real gauge of the quality of her work or the effectiveness of her efforts.

The supervisor, and sometimes the proof-reader, can also provide much the same kind of feedback: number of lines entered, number of errors, deadlines met or quotas reached. Particularly important are opportunities for the data-entry worker herself to provide feedback concerning, for example, handwriting quality or other difficulties, to explain to authors the potential uses and limitations of the equipment being used or to directly discuss and solve problems which arise in the course of work. These activities, however, require communication with colleagues outside the word-processing centre.

It is interesting to note that, although formal instructions describe tasks and routines in detail, they may not necessarily give a very accurate impression of how work is carried out in practice. The organisation of office work is, to a large extent, implicitly defined in the practical knowledge of the various office workers. In other words, the informal aspects of office work contribute to the pattern of information processing which constitutes the working environment of the office. A major result of analysis of office work is summed up as follows: "In an office as it presently operates, the knowledge which is both means and product is dependent on interaction between people for its quality, relevance and appropriateness. These interactions are in turn dependent on social practices."[38]

WORKING TIME

While issues of working time have long been a major focus for both labour legislation and collective bargaining, recent developments have tended to pose these issues in new ways. The length of the working week, for example, is under challenge because of the possible employment-generating effects of reductions in working hours, in addition to demands for greater leisure. This is also true of the length of annual leave and the number of paid public holidays.

With respect to data-entry workers, however, one of the main concerns is for greater flexibility in working time arrangements. Almost all data-entry workers are women, many of whom have family responsibilities. They tend to be young and particularly concerned with the "quality of life". At the same time, the content of their jobs gives them little reason to consider work as having a central role in their lives. They are thus particularly interested in arrangements, such as part-time work, which allow them to adapt their work to their personal lives, rather than the other way round. At the same time, they resist the inflexibility or lack of choice resulting, for example, from compulsory overtime or shift work. Finally, rest pauses are becoming more and more important because of fatigue and stress attributed to working with VDUs.

Normal hours of work

Normal hours of work for data-entry workers tend to be the same as those for clerical and office workers in general. The normal working week of 40 hours spread over five working days (eight hours per day) has been largely achieved in most industrialised countries. Indeed, in some countries (e.g. Canada, the United Kingdom, the United States) a large proportion of office employees work between 35 and 37.5 hours weekly. However, for some workers the 40-hour week norm may be exceeded because of overtime and shift work.

Overtime

Management uses overtime to cope with heavy volumes of work, particularly in the event of mechanical breakdowns, strikes, staff cutbacks, absent workers, seasonal demands or deadlines. In addition, because the cost of hiring, training and providing fringe benefits to additional employees can exceed the cost of overtime premiums, management uses overtime to meet increased demand, especially of a temporary or short-term nature.[39] In some cases, overtime may be used to compensate for inefficiency. For example, a study conducted among record-processing workers in 42 district offices in a federal agency in the United States showed that the less productive offices were using the most overtime and that even with this increased time, their total productivity was lower than in the more efficient units.[40]

In some cases the extent of overtime is widespread. For example, in a survey of 310 EDP establishments covering 10,017 data-entry workers in Japan, overtime work of 5–20 hours a month was common to approximately two-thirds of the establishments.[41]

Using clerical workers as an indicator of the extent of overtime worked by data-entry workers, a United States Department of Labor survey of 56,000 households in May 1979 showed that 12.6 per cent of clerical workers worked extended weeks (41 hours or more).[42] While the number of workers working overtime is low, overtime may be a major inconvenience for those actually affected if long extra hours are required on a specific day or with little notice.

Some collective agreements give the worker the right to refuse overtime. However, even if overtime is not compulsory, it may be the case that the relatively low incomes of most data-entry workers, and their lack of job security, make overtime a necessity.

Shift work

Relatively little information exists about the number of data-entry workers who work on shifts. This could be for two reasons: the general lack of data concerning the extent of shift work in the tertiary or service sector, where most data-entry workers are likely to be found; and the difficulty in isolating data-entry work from the highly diversified jobs found in this sector.

However, there are indications that shift work is being introduced and is in some cases increasing for data-entry work. For example, the major growth area of shift work is among computer operators and related occupations.[43] At the same time, case studies have shown increases in shift work among the data-entry workers they describe.[44]

Part-time employment

Part-time employment is defined as follows in a study prepared by the International Labour Office: "work on a regular and voluntary basis for a daily or weekly period of substantially shorter duration than current normal or statutory hours of work".[45]

Part-time employment is increasing both in absolute terms and as a percentage of total employment. In the early 1980s there were more than 9 million part-time workers throughout the European Community (EC),[46]

13 million in the United States non-agricultural sector alone,[47] 3.9 million in Japan,[48] 1.3 million in Canada[49] and 1 million in Australia.[50] During the same period, part-time workers accounted for approximately 20 per cent of the labour force in the United Kingdom, 16 per cent in Australia, 14.4 per cent in the United States and 10 per cent in Japan.[51]

The vast majority of part-time workers are women, the proportion usually ranging from two-thirds to 90 per cent. Part-time workers also account for a relatively high percentage of total female employment. For example, according to recent figures, the percentage of employed women in part-time employment was 45 per cent in Sweden, 23.6 per cent in the EC in 1979, 23 per cent in the United States and 19.3 per cent in Japan.[52]

A high proportion of part-time women workers are married[53] and are in the childbearing and childrearing age groups.[54] Moreover, a greater proportion of part-time as compared with full-time women workers tend to have dependent children. For example, in the United Kingdom, 70 per cent of women working part time, but only 30 per cent of those working full time, have dependent children.

To what extent are these part-time women workers found in clerical occupations? A 1981 New Earnings Survey of occupational distribution of part-time workers in Great Britain (i.e. the United Kingdom less Northern Ireland) showed that, of all female part-time workers, 23 per cent were clerical.[55] However, it was noted that the survey "under-represents employees (nearly all part-time) earning below the National Insurance deduction cash limit which was £23 a week in the 1981 Survey".[56] The greatest increase in female part-time employment in banking, insurance, finance and business services was associated with the expansion of "other business services" providing employment in secretarial and clerical work. In the United States in 1982, 20.7 per cent (2.9 million out of 14 million) of clerical workers were part-time women workers.[57] In Canada in 1979, 67.1 per cent of part-time opportunities were in sales, service and clerical occupations compared with 36.6 per cent of full-time jobs in these same occupations.[58]

It should be noted that data-entry work lends itself to part-time employment. The work is repetitive and does not require much training nor any real knowledge of office procedures. Moreover, the data-entry task tends to lead quickly to fatigue. Workers may therefore find a full working day too long, while employers may find that hourly productivity is higher for less-fatigued workers. In addition, certain legislative provisions which limit the number of hours per day that can be devoted to data-entry work tend to encourage part-time employment. In particular, it may be difficult for employers to find appropriate tasks to fill the time during the day when data-entry workers are not allowed to work in front of the screen for reasons of health and safety (see below and Chapter 3); it is therefore easier to hire part-time workers who can spend nearly all their working time in front of the VDU.

Rest pauses

A rest pause is a means of overcoming, avoiding or minimising occupationally induced fatigue and stress. It means allowing the data-entry worker to interrupt her work for a period of rest and recovery. Rest pauses are a physiological requirement if performance and efficiency are to be maintained.

Rest pauses are necessary not only during manual work but equally during work that taxes the nervous system, whether by requiring manual dexterity or by the need to monitor a great many incoming sensory inputs. Work at a VDU terminal is particularly tiring and stressful because it requires high concentration and a rapid work pace with virtually no physical activity except operating the keyboard. Consequently, rest pauses are essential to help to avoid some of the effects of fatigue and stress. In this connection, it is significant to note that, although the demand for rest pauses originated from workers' visual discomfort due to intense and extensive VDU viewing and their apprehension concerning its long-term effects, the presence of eye fatigue does not necessarily mean that the source of the problem is actually or purely visual. As some studies have shown, the eye may act as an "early warning system" for the rest of the body.[59]

There is no universally accepted definition of a "pause". A rest pause may be interpreted as a period of inactivity, a specific rest period or an interruption from work or from a specific phase of a task. Studies have shown that people at work take rest pauses of various kinds and under differing circumstances. These include spontaneous pauses (obvious pauses for rest at worker's initiative); disguised pauses (e.g. tidying the work station to relax from her concentration on the main job); work-conditioned pauses (e.g. computer response waiting time or periods of inactivity during machine breakdowns); and prescribed pauses laid down by management (e.g. midday break).

For most VDU work, and particularly for data-entry workers, work-conditioned pauses do not constitute pauses in the sense of rest and recovery. This is particularly true if these waiting times are of unpredictable duration, if they occur during critical stages in the performance of a task and if the workers have no alternative task. For example, during a computer breakdown in an insurance company in Sweden, VDU operators felt "more irritated, tired, rushed and bored . . . than under ordinary working conditions".[60] The situation also led to increases in adrenalin excretion, blood pressure and heart rate. The operators considered machine breakdowns as one of the main sources of stress.

In some countries, legislation and enterprise-level agreements have been formulated to regulate rest pauses. For example, the Ministry of Social Affairs in Austria has issued an ordinance which provides that where work on a VDU is performed for two or more hours without

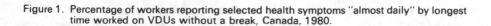

Figure 1. Percentage of workers reporting selected health symptoms "almost daily" by longest time worked on VDUs without a break, Canada, 1980.

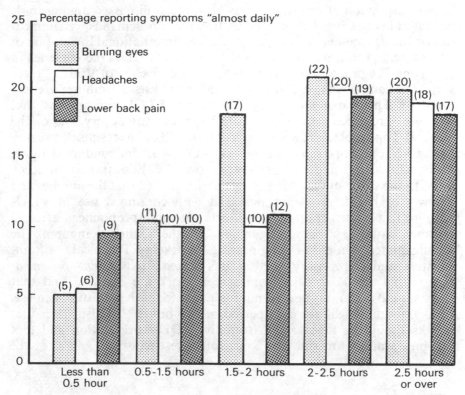

Source: Canadian Labour Congress Labour Education and Studies Centre: *Towards a more humanised technology: Exploring the impact of video display terminals on the health and working conditions of Canadian office workers* (Ottawa, 1982), Appendix I, graph II.

interruption, a break of 10 minutes—to be credited as time worked—is to be included for each 50 minutes of continuous work.[61] In New Zealand, a VDU agreement between the Public Service Association and the State Services Commission provides for a five-minute work break every 30 minutes or a 10-minute work break every hour for VDU operators.[62] In the United Kingdom, numerous technology agreements have been concluded which include provisions concerning rest pauses and VDU work.[63] In some cases, such agreements specify that the rest pause should be taken away from the equipment, preferably in another room where no systems are located.

In the Federal Republic of Germany, VDU operators at an insurance company are protected by an agreement concerning the operating standards for VDUs.[64] The working conditions section of the agreement provides that there must be a 15-minute break after an hour's work and that wherever possible operators will also carry out other tasks which would mean performing a "composite job".

The question of rest pauses has been much discussed among trade unions. This has resulted in various trade union demands, recommendations and guide-lines for negotiations. The International Federation of Commercial, Clerical and Technical Employees (FIET) recommends in its Action Programme that, where there is intensive use of VDUs, "there should be compulsory regular work breaks of at least 10 minutes in every hour".[65] The Canadian Labour Congress (CLC) recommends that workers be required to take 15-minute rest pauses after every hour on the VDU.[66] This recommendation is partially based on the results of a survey on health and working conditions of VDU workers conducted by its Labour Education and Studies Centre (now CLC-Educational Services). Confirming other studies, the survey results showed that the number and severity of health problems increased with continued use of VDUs without rest pauses and that the effects are more pronounced after 90 minutes without a pause (figure 1). In the United Kingdom, the Amalgamated Union of Engineering Workers—Technical, Administrative and Supervisory Section has stated in its *Guide for negotiators* that regular breaks from screen work are essential and that there should preferably be a 10-minute pause for each hour of screen use, or a 20-minute break for each period of two hours.[67] It also states that breaks should be taken away from the VDU work station and that response waiting times do not constitute a rest pause.

Notes

[1] J. Richard Hackman and J. Lloyd Suttle (eds): *Improving life at work: Behavioral science approaches to organizational change* (Santa Monica, California, Goodyear Publishing, 1977), p. 131.

[2] James C. Taylor: *Word processing jobs and organisation: Two case-studies on the quality of working life*, Case-study prepared for the ILO (Geneva, 1979; mimeographed), p. 7.

[3] ibid, pp. 7–8.

[4] M. Lynne Markus: "The new office: More than you bargained for", in *Computerworld*, 23 Feb. 1983, Special issue on "Office Automation", p. 40.

[5] B. Garson: *All the livelong day: The meaning and demeaning of routine work* (Harmondsworth, United Kingdom, Penguin Books, 1977), p. 155.

[6] ILO: "Effects of mechanisation and automation in offices: II", in *International Labour Review*, Mar. 1960, p. 256.

[7] Communications Studies and Planning Ltd.: *Information technology in the office: The impact on women's jobs* (Manchester, Equal Opportunities Commission, 1980), pp. 76–77; Sarah Rolph: "The word is word processing!", in *Datamation* (Los Angeles), Aug. 1979, pp. 124–126.

[8] Piotr Płoszajski et al.: *Characteristics of data-entry jobs in Polish computer centres*, Case study prepared for the ILO (Warsaw, 1979; mimeographed), p. 23.

[9] Communications Studies and Planning Ltd.: *Information technology*; op. cit., p. 79.

[10] Infotech Ltd.: *Office automation: Analysis*, Infotech State of the Art Report, Series 8, No. 3 (Maidenhead, United Kingdom, 1980), p. 116.

[11] Anne Machung: "Turning secretaries into word processors: Some fiction and a fact or two", in Daniel Marschall and Judith Gregory (eds.): *Office automation: Jekyll or Hyde?* (Ohio, Working Women Education Fund, 1983), p. 121.

[12] Leslie Schneider: *Words, words, only words: How word-processing vendors sell their wares in Norway* (Trondheim, Institutt for Industriell Miljøforskning, 1980; mimeographed), p. 6.

[13] ILO: "Effects of mechanisation and automation in offices: II", op. cit., p. 260.

[14] idem: *Problems of women non-manual workers: Work organisation, vocational training, equality of treatment at the workplace, job opportunities*, Report III, Advisory Committee on Salaried Employees and Professional Workers, Eighth Session, Geneva, 1981, p. 63.

[15] Robert Karasek: *A new model of job characteristics and productivity: Relationships between skill underutilization, job stress and low job performance*, Paper prepared for the Conference on Current Issues in Productivity, Columbia University, 18 Apr. 1979 (mimeographed), p. 2.

[16] Rita Kutie: *An analysis of the job dimensions of word-processing secretaries, administrative support secretaries and traditional secretaries, and the correlation of these job dimensions with job satisfaction factors* (unpublished Ph.D. dissertation available in microfilm from University Microfilms International, Ann Arbor, Michigan, and London, 1979), p. 57.

[17] A. M. Young and H. Hayghe: "More US workers are college graduates", in *Monthly Labor Review*, Mar. 1984, p. 46.

[18] Burke D. Grandjean and Patricia A. Taylor: "Job satisfaction among female clerical workers", in *Sociology of Work and Occupations*, Feb. 1980, p. 41.

[19] United States Department of Labor, Bureau of Labor Statistics (BLS): *Educational attainment of workers, March 1979*, Special Labor Force Report 240 (Washington, DC, United States Government Printing Office, 1979), Table J.

[20] Communication Studies and Planning Ltd.: *Information technology . . .* , op. cit., p. 50.

[21] Young and Hayghe, op. cit., p. 48.

[22] Communication Studies and Planning Ltd.: *Information technology . . .* , op. cit., p. 63.

[23] Evelyn Nakano Glenn and Roslyn L. Feldberg: "Degraded and deskilled: The proletarianisation of clerical work", in *Social Problems*, Oct. 1977, p. 57.

[24] See, for example, Enid Mumford and Olive Banks: *The computer and the clerk* (London, Routledge and Kegan Paul, 1967); Leonard Rico: *The advance against paperwork* (Ann Arbor, Michigan, University of Michigan, Bureau of Industrial Relations, 1967), pp. 286–292.

[25] Claudine Marenco: "The effects of the rationalisation of clerical work on the attitudes and behaviour of employees", in Jack Steiber (ed.): *Employment problems of automation and advanced technology* (London, Macmillan, 1966), p. 416.

[26] United Kingdom, Department of Industry: *Microprocessor applications: Cases and observations*, A report prepared by the Massachusetts Institute of Technology (London, 1979), p. 91.

[27] Kay Sykes and Partners Ltd.: *Equal opportunities for secretaries* (London, 1979), cited in Communications Studies and Planning Ltd.: *Information technology . . .* , op. cit., p. 82.

[28] ibid.

[29] Glenn and Feldberg, op. cit., p. 57.

[30] American Management Association: *Establishing an integrated data-processing system*, Special Report No. 11, 1956, p. 113, quoted in Harry Braverman: *Labor and monopoly capital* (New York and London, Monthly Review Press, 1974).

[31] James S. House and James A. Wells: "Occupational stress, social support and health", in: *Reducing occupational stress*, Proceedings of a Conference, Westchester Division, New York Hospital-Cornell Medical Center. 10–12 May, 1977 (Washington, DC, NIOSH, 1978), p. 9.

[32] Michel Crozier: *The bureaucratic phenomenon* (Chicago, University of Chicago Press, 1964), cited in Glenn and Feldberg, op. cit.

[33] See, for example, William L. Renfro: "Second thoughts on moving the office home", in *The Futurist* (Washington, DC), June 1982, pp. 43–48; Labour Canada: *In the chips: Opportunities, people, partnerships*, Report of the Task Force on Micro-electronics and Employment (Ottawa, 1982), p. 57.

[34] An "open-plan" or "open" office design is generally defined as an office with no fixed interior walls or partitions. We use the former term in this book. For more detailed discussion, see Chapter 4.

[35] Greg R. Oldham and Daniel J. Brass: "Employee reactions to an open-plan office: A naturally occurring quasi-experiment", in *Administrative Science Quarterly* (Ithaca, New York), June 1979, pp. 267–283.

[36] Working Women Education Fund: *Warning: Health hazards for office workers* (Cleveland, Ohio, 1981), p. 25.

[37] Glenn and Feldberg, op. cit., p. 62.

[38] E. R. Wynn: *Office conversion as an information medium*, unpublished Ph.D. dissertation (Berkeley, California, 1979), cited in E. Fossum (ed.): *Computerisation of working life* (Chichester, United Kingdom, Ellis Horwood, 1983), p. 134.

[39] United States Department of Labor, BLS: *Long hours and premium pay, May 1978*, Special Labor Force Report 226 (Washington, DC, United States Government Printing Office, 1978), p. 41; Bevars D. Mabry: "The sources of overtime: An integrated perspective", in *Industrial Relations* (Berkeley, California), May 1976, pp. 248–251; George Stamas: "Per cent working long hours shows first post-recession decline", in *Monthly Labor Review*, May 1980, p. 39.

[40] Lloyd S. Baird and Philip J. Beccia: "The potential misuse of overtime", in *Personnel Psychology* (Durham, North Carolina), Autumn 1980, pp. 557–565.

[41] Hajime Saito et al.: *Work-rest schedules and related problems of key operators dealing with computer input data: Results of a survey on 310 establishments*, Case study prepared for the ILO, (Kawasaki, Japan, 1979; mimeographed), p. 14.

[42] United States Department of Labor, BLS: *Long hours and premium pay, May 1979*, Special Labor Force Report 238 (Washington, DC, United States Government Printing Office, 1979).

[43] *Bargaining Report* (London, Labour Research Department), No. 19, Mar.–Apr. 1982, p. 10; European Foundation for the Improvement of Living and Working Conditions: *Shift work in the European Community: The services sector* (Dublin, 1981).

[44] Taylor: *Word processing jobs and organisations*, op. cit., pp. 8, 12; N. De: *Work-system change induced by new technology*, Case study prepared for the ILO (Geneva, 1980; mimeographed), pp. 26–27.

[45] ILO: *Part-time employment: An international survey* (Geneva, doc. ILO/W.4/1973; mimeographed), p. 3.

[46] Eurostat: *Labour Force Sample Survey, 1981*, cited in United Kingdom, House of Lords, Select Committee on the European Communities: *Voluntary part-time work* (London, HMSO, 1982), p. X.

[47] United States Department of Labor, BLS: *Employment and Earnings, April 1982* (Washington, DC, 1982), p. 28.

[48] Japan Institute of Labour: *Problems of working women*, Japanese Industrial Relations Series 8 (Tokyo, 1981), table 6.

[49] Statistics Canada: *Historical labour force statistics, 1979—Actual data, seasonal factors, seasonally adjusted data* (Ottawa, 1980), p. 51.

[50] Mary Beasley: "Permanent part-time work", in John Wilkes (ed.): *The future of work* (Sydney, George Allen and Unwin, 1981), p. 100.

[51] *Department of Employment Gazette* (London), Oct. 1981, p. S. 11, cited in United Kingdom, House of Lords, Select Committee on the European Communities: *Voluntary part-time work*, op. cit., p. ix. Beasley, loc. cit.; United States Department of Labor, BLS: *Employment and Earnings*, loc. cit.; Japan Institute of Labour: *Problems of working women*, loc. cit.

[52] ILO: *Record of Proceedings*, Governing Body, 211th Session, Geneva, 13–16 Nov. 1979 (doc. GB211/2/1), para. 56; Japan Institute of Labour: *Problems of working women*, loc. cit.

[53] ILO: *Record of Proceedings*, loc. cit.; see also James E. Long and Ethel B. Jones: "Married women in part-time employment", in *Industrial and Labor Relations Review* (Ithaca, New York), Apr. 1981, pp. 413–425; Jennifer Hurstfield: *The part-time trap* (London, Low Pay Unit, 1978); Carol Leon and Robert W. Bednarzik: "A profile of women on part-time schedules", in *Monthly Labor Review*, Oct. 1978, pp. 3–12; OPCS: *Labour Force Survey, 1981*, cited in United Kingdom, House of Lords, Select Committee on the European Communities: *Voluntary part-time work*, op. cit., p. XI; Japan Institute of Labour: *Problems of working women*, op. cit., p. 12.

[54] Colin Leicester: "Towards a fully part-time Britain", in *Personnel Management* (London), June 1982, p. 29; United States Department of Labor, BLS: *Handbook of Labor Statistics, 1980* (Washington, DC, Dec. 1980), 23, p. 55.

[55] *New Earnings Survey, 1981*, tables 28 and 138, cited in United Kingdom, House of Lords, Select Committee on the European Communities: *Voluntary part-time work*, op cit., p. XVII.

[56] ibid.

[57] United States Department of Labor, BLS: *Employment and Earnings*, op. cit., table A-30, p. 30.

[58] Canadian Advisory Council on the Status of Women: *Part-time work: A review of the issue*, A brief to the Advisory Council of Employment and Immigration Canada (Ottawa, 1980), p. 4.

[59] A. Cakir et al.: *Visual display terminals*. (Chichester, United Kingdom, John Wiley, 1979), p. 208.

[60] Gunn Johansson and Gunnar Aronsson: *Stress reactions in computerised administrative work* (Stockholm, University of Stockholm, Department of Psychology, 1980), p. 36, reprinted in *Journal of Occupational Behaviour* (Chichester, United Kingdom), July 1984, pp. 159–181.

[61] *OGB-Nachrichtendienst* (Vienna), No. 2137, 11 June 1982, cited in *Social and Labour Bulletin* (Geneva, ILO), No. 3/82, p. 386.

[62] *PSA and SSC VDU Agreement*, Agreement between the Public Service Association and the State Services Commission of New Zealand (mimeographed).

[63] *Bargaining Report*, No. 22, Special issue on Survey of New Technology, pp. 14–15.

[64] *Agreement concerning the installation of video display units within the Volksfürsorge* (Hamburg, Insurance Co-operative Company, June 1979).

[65] International Federation of Commercial, Clerical and Technical Employees (FIET): *Computers and work: FIET Action Programme* (Geneva, 1979), p. 16.

[66] Canadian Labour Congress (CLC) Labour Education and Studies Centre: *Towards a more humanized technology: Exploring the impact of video display terminals on the health and working conditions of Canadian office workers* (Ottawa, 1982), p. 166.

[67] United Kingdom, Amalgamated Union of Engineering Workers—Technical, Administrative and Supervisory Section (AUEW-TASS): *New technology—A guide for negotiators: A policy statement by TASS* (London, 1978), cited in European Trade Union Institute (ETUI): *Redesigning jobs: Western European experiences* (Brussels, 1981), p. 140.

HEALTH, SAFETY AND ERGONOMIC ASPECTS OF DATA-ENTRY WORKPLACES

3

Much has been said and written recently about the health, safety and ergonomic aspects of VDU workplaces. In this chapter, some issues and problems are examined which relate to the working environment (e.g. lighting, noise, ventilation and humidity) and VDU work station (e.g. screens, keyboards, furniture). Of course, to a large extent the nature and organisation of the task itself influences the effects of these factors. This chapter also indicates the impact these factors can have in terms of symptoms among workers. However, problems concerning occupational stress are discussed in Chapter 4.

THE WORKING ENVIRONMENT

This section describes certain features of the working environment—such as lighting, noise, ventilation and humidity—which have important effects on workers' safety, health, comfort and effectiveness. Many of these features are treated in general analyses of occupational safety and health in offices. However, the discussion below emphasises those points which have been of particular concern for data-entry work. It is assumed that the work is taking place in an office or similar workplace.

Lighting

The most important feature of the working environment involved in the interaction between a data-entry worker and a VDU is lighting conditions in the room. In some cases, lighting will have been determined without specific consideration of the VDU. Some data-entry operators work in areas which are often described as "twilight" or semi-darkness, while others suffer from glare or excessive brightness. In the United States, for example, a National Institute for Occupational Safety and Health (NIOSH) study of VDU operators in clerical jobs showed that while the illumination levels were generally in the 500–700 lux range, levels as low as 300 lux and as high as 1,200 lux were also observed.[1] Optimum lighting conditions at VDU workplaces depend on several factors, such as the characteristics of the screen, the keyboard, the viewing angle (e.g. positioning vis-à-vis windows and light fixtures) and the nature of the visual task. Illumination levels tend to be somewhat higher for data-entry terminal workplaces than for conversational or dialogue terminal workplaces. Data-entry workers adjust their lighting conditions in such a way as to allow good reading of source documents, while operators on conversational terminals choose good reading conditions on the screen.[2] When viewing, operators prefer low levels of illumination to avoid or minimise reflection from the screen.[3] This is likely to induce visual strain as the data-entry operator switches between viewing the source document and the screen. It should be noted that, for data-entry operators, the length of uninterrupted looks at either source documents or the screen is much shorter than for conversational or dialogue terminal operators, and thus the frequency of sweeping glances is much higher for the data-entry group.[4]

In addition, some studies have indicated that the glare from fluorescent strip lighting in areas where VDU screens are in use has contributed to worker discomfort.

Noise

While VDUs are quieter than typewriters, their cooling fans or transformers still hum and whirr. Even if the level of this kind of noise is low, the frequency and continuous exposure can be irritating or obtrusive to some operators, particularly those with a high sensitivity to high-frequency noise and whose task requires concentration. In general, however, noise problems at VDU workplaces are caused by printers.

The noise of keypunching machines is more of a problem.[5] The steady clatter which accompanies the preparation of cards is reported to contribute to worker fatigue, nervous tension and lower productivity.

Ventilation and humidity

Temperature problems in VDU workplaces depend on, among other things, the power consumption of the equipment, the room lighting and the number of people in the room. VDUs emit heat during their operation. This imposes an additional thermal load, which the heating and ventilation system may not have been designed to handle. In a survey in which a sample of 1,021 VDU operators were asked if they felt that the air temperature in the room was pleasant or otherwise, less than 25 per cent found the air temperature to be satisfactory or better.[6] Usually when there are several units in a room, "the combined thermal emission from the

VDUs is sufficient to raise the average temperature in the room, often in spite of ventilation".[7] Sometimes the units in the room are poorly arranged and the heat emitted by a VDU is directed towards neighbouring operators.

Relative humidity is another component of the working environment which is important as regards the comfort of the operator at work. In most offices, the air tends to be too dry. This leads to drying of the mucous membranes of the eyes and nose, which increases the risk of infection. In the above-mentioned survey, between 70 and 95 per cent of those interviewed judged the air in the room as too dry.[8]

A related ventilation problem concerns air circulation. Many office workers complain of draughts, particularly in the region of the neck, shoulders, back and legs. For example, more than half of those questioned in the previously mentioned survey complained about the effects of draughts around the legs and neck. On the other hand, in some cases, "sealed" older buildings and newly constructed "energy-efficient" buildings may mean an inadequate supply of fresh air. This can produce headaches and drowsiness, and can interfere with concentration.

THE DATA-ENTRY WORK STATION

The data-entry work station consists of equipment and furniture that the operator uses during the execution of her tasks. The most important components are the VDU screen, the keyboard and office furniture. The problems associated with these factors obviously interact. However, in order to understand the nature of these problems, we examine the different aspects separately.

The VDU screen

The visual display or screen provides the operator with a means— and often the only means—for checking the content and accuracy of the information she is entering or for searching in order to locate certain information, errors, and so on. Screen characteristics have been widely implicated as a major source of workers' physical discomfort. These characteristics or properties include—

(a) the contrast between the background (screen) and the characters;

(b) the legibility of the characters;

(c) the display capacity of the screen (size of screen and number of characters displayed);

(d) image stability ("flickering" of the image);

(e) the colour of the screen; and

(f) the presence of parasitic sources of light on the screen itself.

Moreover, some of these likely problem sources, particularly in conjunction with reflections from windows and overhead lighting, can lead to or exacerbate glare for the operator. For example, in the NIOSH study mentioned above, reflected glare was present in most of the VDU screens surveyed, and most of the operators found glare, screen and character brightness, flicker and illegibility "bothersome".[9]

Some observers note that the problems concerning light and VDU screens are made more complicated by technological limitations.[10] These relate to the brightness level of characters with respect to normal room lighting, and glare problems which are exacerbated as a result of the necessary screen curvature and the position and angle chosen by the operators as most comfortable.

There has also been some controversy concerning the cathode ray or ionising and non-ionising radiation emitted by VDUs. Since VDU design is based on the application of cathode ray tube (CRT) technology, it is inevitable that certain types of radiation are generated. Ultraviolet, visible and infra-red radiation are emitted by the phosphor material when stimulated by the electron beam within the CRT; X-rays may also be generated, as with the CRT in a television receiver; and radio frequency (RF) radiation may be produced by some of the electronic components and circuits.[11] Nevertheless, over time, there have been improvements in design which have resulted in lower levels of radiation. Some studies have found, for example, that RF levels drop off rapidly with distance from the source and that measured levels were much lower than the most stringent standards set anywhere in the world.[12]

A related area of controversy which has recently attracted attention concerns reports of abnormal pregnancies (miscarriages, premature births, birth defects) said to be linked with the use of VDUs. The most commonly suggested cause is radiation, even though radiation emission from the unit tested has been either non-detectable or many times lower than the currently accepted occupational health limit. Research is currently in progress concerning the possible effects of varying levels of radiation and duration of exposure, with particular emphasis on the long-term effects of exposure to low-level radiation. A complicating factor is that abnormal pregnancies can be related to many factors other than radiation exposure, both at home and at work.

At present, there is no consensus that there is any direct causal relationship between radiation and these occurrences. Meanwhile, until the results of more comprehensive research are available, various preventive measures to protect VDU workers from any potential reproductive hazards have been proposed or introduced in many workplaces. These include assigning vulnerable persons to non-VDU work, regular rest pauses, limited total time of VDU use per day, and periodic testing and regular maintenance of VDUs. Other measures relate to minimising or eliminating the stress-inducing features of some jobs (see Chapters 4 and 5).

The keyboard

Certain keyboard characteristics can pose problems which aggravate the fatigue and discomfort of the operator. Some of these characteristics are keyboard thickness and height, colour and reflection of the keys and the keyboard surfaces, keyboard layout and feedback, key force, and size and coding of key legends. The development of the detachable or movable keyboard, however, has alleviated some of the fatigue experienced by the operator.

It should be noted that, while the VDU keyboard is similar to the alphanumeric keyboard on a conventional typewriter, it is a more complex instrument. The keyboard itself has one or more sets of function keys and perhaps also an auxiliary numeric set of keys in addition to the main alphanumeric key set. Moreover, greater care is required in the use of the function and command keys, particularly those of which inadvertent operation may result in serious consequences. This is due to the fact that the VDU is part of a system wherein the flow and manipulation of information take a more abstract form compared with the tangible piece of paper in a typewriter.

It should also be noted that many of the features of VDU and typewriter keyboards are a direct result of design decisions that were made to overcome purely mechanical limitations of the time. For example, the relative placings or positions of the characters in the QWERTY keyboard layout were not, as is commonly believed, chosen for the convenience of the operator but for reasons associated with the construction of the type bar mechanism in mechanical typewriters. The QWERTY keyboard layout has become, with minor national variations, the universal keyboard layout, and its persistence today is largely the result of habit and custom rather than attention to sound ergonomic principles. For instance, one of the criticisms levelled at the QWERTY keyboard layout is that, "in English-language typing, about 60 per cent of the workload is carried by the left hand which, for most of the population, is the non-preferred hand".[13] Moreover, the frequent use of capital letters in some languages (e.g. in German) requires frequent use of the shift key, which results in greater physiological loading of the little fingers than is necessary when typing texts, for example, in English or French.

Furniture and work station configuration

Poorly designed furniture has major implications for the worker's comfort, safety and health, and efficiency. Many symptoms of physical fatigue, neck, shoulder or back pains, as well as visual discomfort or eye strain, can also be attributed to such factors: desks that are too high or too low; chairs that are rigid or unadjustable or that are too high or too low, or with no backrests; cramped work stations (e.g. inadequate leg room); no footrests to correct leg posture for smaller persons; and no document holders to avoid an unfavourable inclination of the head. In the previously mentioned NIOSH survey, placing VDU terminals on standard office desks resulted, in some cases, in keyboards that were higher than optimum for any but relatively tall operators, while in some cases the VDU screen heights were too low for a tall operator.[14] In all the work stations examined, the minimum keyboard and screen heights were set by the design of the non-adjustable furniture. In a few cases, however, the keyboard was raised by the operator by, for example, placing stacks of newspapers under the keyboard.

It is interesting to note that operators sometimes believe that these parameters are fixed and thus do not realise that they could be changed. In other cases, although the furniture is adjustable, the operators do not know how to make adjustments. Moreover, even if the furniture or the work station is ergonomically well designed, this is no guarantee against fatigue. For example, if the job itself requires the operator to maintain a static position or permits only a few essential movements, the most "ergonomically correct" or the "most desirable" sitting posture will soon become fatiguing.

EFFECTS ON THE WORKER OF POORLY DESIGNED WORK STATIONS

It has become increasingly clear in recent years that office and data-entry work involves health and safety problems. The introduction of mechanised technology has exacerbated old problems and added some new ones. There is a fairly large body of evidence documenting the presence of a wide range of physical and psychological symptoms among VDU workers. According to Ostberg, who has carried out comprehensive studies in this area, operators who use VDUs suffer from a wide range of alarming symptoms ranging from mere discomfort to pain and extreme visual fatigue. These include eye strain, visual deterioration, headaches and changes in normal visual acuity. In some cases, operators reported changes in colour perception, a dulling of sensation in the fingertips, temperature and noise discomfort from the equipment, extreme stress and fatigue, and dissatisfaction with their work.[15]

These symptoms are not caused by a single factor through a simple chain of events. Work environment factors interact with each other, and with task demands and social and psychological aspects of the work. It is rarely possible to attribute any specific effect or symptom to an individual cause. For this reason, studies on the health, safety and comfort of data-entry workers concentrate on symptoms found among the workers and attempt to identify the multiple causes of these symptoms. The most important of these symptoms are eye strain and visual problems, postural discomfort and occupational stress.

In this section, symptoms related to eye strain and visual problems and postural discomfort are examined separately, although they are obviously related. Moreover, symptoms of physiological discomfort and fatigue can contribute to psychological stress. However, the topic of occupational stress is complex and requires a separate analysis. It is therefore discussed in Chapter 4.

Visual discomfort

The most common complaint among data-entry workers using VDUs concerns visual discomfort, or what is loosely described as "eye-strain". More specifically, such complaints refer to symptoms such as burning eyes, watery eyes, red eyes, shooting pains, twitching eye muscles and dry eyes. Other reported symptoms relate to visual impairment, such as blurring or difficulty in focusing on objects near or far, flicker vision and seeing colour fringes or double images. Headaches are the most common general symptom, but the operator may not always connect the headache with eye-strain.

In a field study of office workers performing different tasks (data-entry terminals, conversational terminals, traditional office work and typing), it was shown that visual impairment was more frequent in VDU operators.[16] Moreover, this impairment persisted frequently until sleeping time and some operators avoided watching television or reading during their leisure time.

A survey of 2,336 office workers in 15 workplaces across Canada revealed a higher incidence of eye-strain and visual problems in VDU users compared with non-VDU users.[17] Moreover, workers whose jobs required the intensive use of VDUs, such as those in "production line" (e.g. reservation agents) and "data-entry" categories, reported substantially greater numbers of and more severe health problems than other workers.

Another survey carried out by the London-based Alfred Marks Bureau showed that "eye-strain is the most common complaint of VDU operators, and headaches and migraines are suffered most often by data preparation staff".[18]

In France, a survey carried out by the *Institut national de recherche et de sécurité* (INRS) compared a group of data-entry operators with a group of "interactive" operators (using the computer in dialogue or question-and-answer mode). One of the major results of the study was a higher rate of visual disorder among the former (50–60 per cent) than the latter (30–40 per cent), although the total proportion of working time spent looking at the screen represented only 15–25 per cent for data-entry workers, as against 30–40 per cent in the case of the dialogue system.[19]

The symptoms of eye-strain and visual fatigue may be caused or aggravated by a number of different factors. One set of factors relates to the characteristics of the VDU workplace and of the job. These factors include—

(a) the design characteristics of the keyboard (e.g. matt or glossy keys, thin or thick keyboard, fixed or detachable keyboard), the screen (e.g. character size, legibility, spacing), the furniture (e.g. adjustable chairs and desks) and the overall work station configuration;

(b) the nature, content or type of VDU task (task requirements) and the organisation of the working procedure, such as duration of uninterrupted working periods, degree of concentration required, freedom to pause at will and the use of source documents; and

(c) the characteristics of the working environment, such as the level of illumination, the effects of reflecting surfaces (windows, desks, office decoration), the availability of daylight and artificial lighting, and the amount of ventilation and noise.[20]

Another set of factors which could influence the likelihood and severity of visual fatigue concerns the personal characteristics of the operator. These include the incidence of eyesight defects in operators, age, working posture and constitutional factors such as poor health and tiredness.

"Perfect vision" is rare, and it has been shown that visual fatigue occurs or is magnified if the worker is already suffering from uncorrected or improperly corrected eye defects. Moreover, visual performance gradually deteriorates throughout adult life, and this decrease is especially marked between the ages of 30 and 50. The more common types of visual disorders are long-sightedness (hypermetropia), short-sightedness (myopia), astigmatism and accommodation problems due to age. These common disorders are often compensated for by the use of eyeglasses or corneal contact lenses. However, these may pose problems in using VDUs. Prescription lenses for "reading glasses" are normally ground for script reading at 30 cm from the eye, while lenses for "distant" viewing are usually ground at 200 cm or more. VDU operators usually view the screen at distances between 50 and 70 cm and the keyboard at about 45–50 cm. This means that the use of prescription lenses may create "out-of-focus" problems.

Visual acuity may not be the sole factor, however. It has been noted that with work involving a display screen the eye has constantly to adapt its focus, since it must continually move from the screen to the keyboard or to the reference document, each of which is located at a different distance. Moreover, it is well known that "keeping the eye perfectly still in order to aim at a target is very demanding on it, and that consequently eye strain is not due solely to the movement of the eye but also to the effort involved in keeping it still".[21] This process of accommodation or adaptation may pose particular problems for older workers. For example, they may attempt to overcome the problem by trying to reduce the visual distance by changing posture, but then this leads to fatigue in the neck and back.

The situation is often aggravated for those workers who use bifocal glasses, since they must adopt a fatiguing head posture which often leads to excessive tension in the neck and even pinched nerves in the upper spine.

The symptoms of visual fatigue described above—burning eyes, watery eyes, double vision, etc.—are reversible. After a short period of rest, these symptoms recede and normal vision returns. Tests on long-term or irreversible effects are inconclusive, and the possibility of irreversible effects is not supported on the basis of current medical experience. "This does not mean to say, however, that such a possibility and, perhaps more importantly, individual anxieties concerning such a possibility should not be taken seriously."[22] Moreover, it should be emphasised that, while fatigue among VDU workers may be experienced as various symptoms of visual discomfort, the source of the problem need not necessarily be visual. Visual symptoms do not necessarily imply a purely visual problem; as previously noted, the eyes may act as an "early warning system" for the rest of the body.

Postural discomfort

Data-entry workers using VDUs also suffer from musculo-skeletal problems. In the previously mentioned survey of Canadian office workers, VDU operators (particularly data-entry workers) experienced a significantly higher incidence of neck, shoulder and arm pains.[23] Another study undertaken by Hünting et al., of the Department of Hygiene and Ergonomics of the Swiss Federal Institute of Technology in Zurich, found that among data-entry terminal operators a larger proportion (60 per cent) suffered from sore shoulders than among conversational terminal operators (30 per cent), non-VDU typists (25 per cent) or non-VDU traditional office workers (10 per cent).[24]

Earlier studies concerning keypunch operators revealed that they also suffered from physical pains in the hands, neck, shoulders and arms.[25]

The probable causes of postural discomfort, like the causes of visual discomfort, are manifold and inter-related. These causes relate to the static or fixed working position, the nature and organisation of the task, matching posture to the visual task, equipment design and the working environment.

Postural immobilisation has considerable influence on feelings of fatigue by data-entry workers. The human body is designed for movement, and static loads imposed by constant sitting are more tiring than the loads imposed by movement. Most data-entry workers at VDU work stations, often limited to operating the terminal, remain in the same working position for long uninterrupted periods of time. It is important to note that such a work station, which requires the worker to maintain a single so-called "optimum" posture, cannot really be considered an "optimum" work station. To a large extent, this static position is determined by the nature of the task. The task itself requires or allows only a minimum of body movements. Moreover, these body movements associated with the task may themselves be a source of loading and fatigue. The data-entry task requires only the frequently repeated movements of certain parts of the body (e.g. hands, neck) during relatively long periods of time.

Data-entry work is often considered as repetitive and lacking in variety. Studies have shown that with "increasing repetitiveness in the work, the frequency of all types of complaint increases markedly".[26] For example, in a survey of more than 1,000 VDU operators in different jobs, those with the most "one-sided" types of activity (i.e. input copy typists or data-entry operators) experienced more frequent pains in the back and sought orthopaedic treatment more frequently than any other category of clerical worker using VDUs.[27] Analysis of the frequency of postural complaints among different groups of VDU users indicate that—

(a) the physiological demands on VDU operators are highly dependent on the nature of their jobs;

(b) the same demands tend to decrease with work that is less repetitive; and

(c) those VDU operators whose jobs are of a varied nature and who are not bound to remain at their workplace are the least likely to suffer postural discomfort.[28]

Postural discomfort often occurs when the operator performs VDU task activities such as looking at source documents, the display screen or keyboard, operating the keyboard and working with source documents. In doing this, the operator may assume a posture which ultimately leads to discomfort and pain. For example, certain movements (e.g. bending the head and upper part of the body to view the screen, keyboard and source documents; sideways movement and twisting in looking from the screen or keyboard towards the document; and bending and stretching when alternately viewing the screen and keyboard) can place loading on different parts of the spinal column.[29]

Equipment design, particularly of the visual screen and the keyboard, can influence the working posture of VDU operators. If the display is difficult to read because, for example, the characters are too small or the contrast too low, the operator will be inclined to lean forward. If the screen has specular reflections, the operator will move her head in such a way that reflection is minimised or avoided. This, among other things, can result in an inclined and uncomfortable position.

The characteristics of the keyboard can also lead to poor working posture. The VDU keyboard is usually operated with the hands and arms in an unsupported position. This often leads to fatigue and ailments in the shoulder/arm region. The situation is often aggravated by the sunken keyboard (i.e. the keyboard as an integral part of the VDU chassis), where there is a small and insufficient space to rest the hands.

Keyboard thickness and the height of the keyboard from the floor also have important implications for the operator experiencing fatigue in the neck, arms and back. Keyboards that are too high or too thick force the operator to assume an awkward position in order to read the source document or the screen. Studies have shown that there is a relationship between such complaints and the height of the keyboard surface: with those using data-entry terminals which were higher than the average of 7–8 cm, more pains in hands and arms were reported.

The colour and reflectability characteristics of the keys and keyboard are also closely related to operators' fatigue and muscular discomfort. For example, complaints of fatigue are twice as frequent among VDU operators who use machines with glossy black keys as among operators with lighter-coloured, matt-finished keyboards.[30]

With regard to office furniture, chairs, backrests and desks which are not adjustable to suit the anthropometric characteristics of the worker and the requirements of the data-entry task oblige the operator to assume an awkward position which leads to stiffening of the muscles of the shoulders, arms and back and to neck pains resulting from constant turning.

Finally, the quality of the source document may also contribute to postural discomfort. There is a relationship between the legibility of the document and working posture. For example, a text that is handwritten in pencil tends to become difficult to read at large viewing angles because of glare, with the result that the worker continually tries to find a position in which reading ability is improved. Usually she will find it necessary to bend over the document and to twist the head sideways to reduce the viewing distance. Working in this position for long periods of time obviously leads to fatigue. The use of carbon duplicates and photocopies also leads to similar problems. Moreover, the different luminance of the source document and the keyboard requires longer visual accommodation and pupil adjustment than would be the case if they had the same luminance. This may have an influence on the posture of the operator and the likelihood of postural and visual discomfort.

Working environment conditions, such as lighting and ventilation, can also add to postural loading problems. For example, room illumination levels which are too high, or reflections from windows, light fixtures and furniture, for example, may force the worker to assume an awkward posture to minimise glare.

Finally, it is important to bear in mind that there is no single perfect workplace design nor a single "ergonomic" VDU work station. Different user and task characteristics generate their own specific requirements. Consequently, no uniform guide-lines can be established for all types of VDU workplaces.[31] However, based on available research, it is possible to formulate recommendations for good practice. For the reasons explained, most guide-lines for VDU workplace design contain a certain degree of flexibility.[32] Most of these indicate a range of values and characteristics which permits the operator to design, or have designed for her, a workplace that best meets her needs.

Notes

[1] L. Stammerjohn et al.: "Evaluation of work station design factors in VDT operations", in *Human Factors* (Santa Monica, California), Aug. 1981, pp. 401–412.

[2] Th. Läubli et al.: "Visual impairments of VDU operators related to environmental conditions", in E. Grandjean and E. Vigliani (eds.): *Ergonomic aspects of visual display terminals* (London, Taylor and Francis, 1980), pp. 85–94.

[3] Houshang Shahnavaz: "Lighting conditions and workplace dimensions of VDU operators", in *Ergonomics* (London), Dec. 1982, pp. 1165–1173.

[4] R. Elias et al.: "Investigations in operators working with CRT display terminals: Relationships between task content and psychophysiological alterations", in Grandjean and Vigliani, op. cit., pp. 211–217.

[5] ILO: "Effects of mechanisation and automation in offices: III", in *International Labour Review*, Apr. 1960, p. 351; Ida Russakoff Hoos: "The impact of office automation on workers", in *International Labour Review*, Oct. 1960, pp. 363–388.

[6] A. Cakir et al.: *Visual display terminals* (Chichester, John Wiley, 1980), p. 225.

[7] ibid.

[8] ibid., p. 222.

[9] Stammerjohn et al., op. cit., p. 8.

[10] B. Morton: "Display eye strain: A manufacturer's view", in *Computing Europe*, 12 July 1979, pp. 14–15.

[11] Cakir et al., op. cit., pp. 23–25; T. Terrana et al.: "Electromagnetic radiations emitted by visual display units", in Grandjean and Vigliani, op. cit., pp. 13–21.

[12] United States, Bureau of Radiological Health: *An evaluation of radiation emissions from visual display terminals*, HHS Publication FDA 81-8153 (Rockville, Maryland, United States Department of Health and Human Services, Food and Drug Administration, 1981).

[13] Cakir et al., op. cit., p. 137.

[14] Stammerjohn et al., op. cit., p. 8.

[15] O. Ostberg: "CRTs pose health problems for operators", in *Health and Safety* (London), Nov.–Dec. 1975.

[16] Th. Läubli et al.: "Postural and visual loads at VDT workplaces: II. Lighting conditions and visual impairments", in *Ergonomics*, Dec. 1981, pp. 933–944.

[17] CLC Labour Education and Studies Centre: *Towards a more humanised technology: Exploring the impact of video display terminals on the health and working conditions of Canadian office workers* (Ottawa, 1982).

[18] A. Thomas: "Operators are bored and troubled by office technology, says report", in *Computer Weekly*, 11 Feb. 1982, p. 13, with reference to Alfred Marks Bureau, Statistical Services Division: *The machine dream: A report on the experience and expectations of companies employing full-time machine operators to improve office productivity* (London, n.d.).

[19] R. Elias and F. Cail: *Constraintes et astreintes devant les terminaux à écran cathodique*, Report No. 1189/RE (Paris, Institut national de recherche et de sécurité, 1982).

[20] Cakir et al., op. cit., p. 209; J. Crespy and P. Rey: *Work on visual display units: Risks for health*, Paper prepared for the World Health Organization (Geneva, doc. WHO/OCH/83.2; mimeographed); B. Brown et al.: "Video display terminals and vision of workers", in *Behaviour and Information Technology* (London and Philadelphia), Vol. 1, No. 2, 1982, pp. 121–140.

[21] ILO: *The effects of technological and structural changes on the employment and working conditions of non-manual workers*, Report II, Advisory Committee on Salaried Employees and Professional Workers, Eighth Session, Geneva, 1981 (Geneva, 1980), p. 99.

[22] Cakir et al., op. cit., p. 215.

[23] CLC Labour Education and Studies Centre: *Towards a more humanised technology . . .* , op. cit.

[24] W. Hünting et al.: "Constrained postures of VDU operators", in Grandjean and Vigliani, op. cit. p. 179, figure 2; idem.: "Postural and visual loads at VDT workplaces: I. Constrained postures", in *Ergonomics*, Dec. 1981, pp. 917–931.

[25] Y. Komoike and S. Hariguchi: "Fatigue assessment on keypunch operators, typists and others", in K. Hashimoto et al. (eds.): *Methodology in human fatigue assessment* (London, Taylor and Francis, 1971), pp. 101–110; ILO: "Effects of mechanisation and automation in offices: III", in *International Labour Review*, Apr. 1960, pp. 350–369.

[26] Cakir et al., op. cit., p. 197.

[27] ibid., p. 245.

[28] ibid., p. 197.

[29] Hünting et al.: "Constrained posture of VDU operators", op. cit.

[30] Cakir et al., op. cit., p. 202–203.

[31] E. Grandjean: "Ergonomics of VDUs: Review of present knowledge", in Grandjean and Vigliani op. cit., p. 10; Shahnavaz, op. cit.

[32] See, for example, Cakir et al., op. cit.; E. Grandjean et al.: "Preferred VDT work station settings, body posture and physical impairments", in *Applied Ergonomics* (Surrey, Butterworth), June 1984, pp. 99–104; Wilbert O. Galitz: *Human factors in office automation* (Atlanta, Georgia, Life Office Management Association, 1980), pp. 183–197.

DATA-ENTRY WORK AND OCCUPATIONAL STRESS

4

In Chapters 2 and 3, the need for improvement in several characteristics of data-entry jobs was discussed, with emphasis on work organisation, working time and occupational health, safety and ergonomics. The justification for such improvements is usually to overcome specific problems which face data-entry workers. These problems are all-important and deserve separate attention. Moreover, the interaction among them is critical to understanding their overall impact. This chapter, therefore, considers the ways that these specific problems can interact and produce a combination of effects on data-entry workers.

It is by now widely recognised that a job can be inappropriate and damaging to the worker without there being any obvious immediate physical harm. A wide variety of concepts have been proposed as capturing some of the social, psychological and physical factors involved: alienation, anomy, anxiety, boredom, conflict, fatigue, frustration, job satisfaction (and dissatisfaction), overload, pressure, and so on. These concepts, defined and measured in many different ways, have in turn been investigated in terms of their outcomes for both the enterprise and the individual: absenteeism, turnover, poor work quality, low productivity, health of the worker, and so forth.

In recent years, increased attention has been paid to occupational stress as a concept which has many advantages in investigating the quality or appropriateness of work, especially from the viewpoint of worker protection.[1] These advantages include the following:

(1) The concept of stress offers ways of combining seemingly disparate factors concerning characteristics of jobs and the working environment (e.g. physical work environment, social climate, work content) and effects on workers (e.g. absenteeism, apathy, neurosis, ulcers) into a coherent analytical framework.

(2) Stress can be measured, at least partly, in terms of "hard" medical evidence (e.g. substances in blood or urine) instead of merely by "soft" sociological or psychological techniques.

(3) The symptoms of stress include health problems (cardio-vascular disease, gastro-intestinal disorders, depression, neuroses, etc.) which demand serious attention.

In addition, the empirical evidence on stress has been particularly convincing as regards the effects of mechanisation and computerisation. As will be seen below, it lends itself especially well to an analysis of the very problems most frequently confronted by data-entry workers.

On the other hand, it must be admitted that occupational stress remains a complex, controversial topic. The many definitions and models of stress that exist are designed to meet specific needs for different types of research. It seems unlikely that a single definition can meet all these needs at this time. A framework which includes the main characteristics of most of these definitions has the following essential features, dividing the stress syndrome into its elements or interacting processes:

(a) the sources of stress in the physical work environment and the organisation of work;

(b) the individual differences among workers which condition, or moderate their perception of, vulnerability and responses to potential sources of stress; and

(c) the effects of stress.

The sources or causes of stress at work are often associated with the physical work environment (e.g. noise, glare), equipment design (e.g. monitoring devices, high screen luminance) and organisational factors (e.g. work overload, close supervision). These sources of stress are often inter-related and mutually reinforcing.

The transition or the path from potential sources of stress in the work environment to consequences for the health and well-being of workers is influenced by the characteristics of the individual. Individual vulnerability to specific job-related sources of stress is complex and varies widely for each person, as well as for different persons. These individual differences (e.g. age, family responsibilities, qualifications) are critical factors in experiencing and responding to occupational stress.

The effects of work stress—i.e. the consequences for the individual—can be physiological (e.g. increase in heart rate), psychological (e.g. depression, anxiety) and behavioural (e.g. increased error rates). Stress has been shown to be both a "disease producer" and a "disease enhancer". Moreover—

In relation to illness, stress can play a *direct* role—as with ulcers or coronary heart disease—an *additional* role—aggravating diabetes, asthma, cancer or skin rashes—or a *synergistic* role—creating a combined health risk greater than two or more problems simply added together, as in the case of someone who smokes and is under stress.[2]

Finally, some stress is healthy, in so far as demands on the worker can be perceived as a challenge (e.g. the opportunity to do a more complex job) rather than a constraint (e.g. excessive pace, monotonous task). It is intense, continuous or prolonged stress—chronic stress—which endangers physical and mental health.[3]

MYTHS ABOUT STRESS AT WORK

Recent research findings contradict commonly held ideas about stress. These findings surprised many people when they revealed the high levels of stress endured by clerical and secretarial workers. It disproved the popular belief that people who have great responsibilities and who make many important decisions are the ones who experience the most stress. One factor which partly accounts for some of the astonishment is that before the 1970s most stress research was carried out on white males only and focused on "executive" or "managerial" stress, particularly in terms of their susceptibility to coronary heart disease (CHD). A myth has grown up that managers are the group most "at risk" in this respect.

The new findings also disprove commonly heard ideas such as that stress comes from the home (personal and family problems) and is carried into work, or that stress is "an individual sort of thing" and has nothing to do with the job. Findings clearly indicate that conditions of work and the characteristics of jobs may be powerful sources of stress. For example, research in the United States and Europe shows that one of the major determinants of stress is lack of control over the content and pace of work. Moreover, stress experienced by the worker on the job lasts much longer than the hours spent at the workplace. Stress at work is "taken home" and affects relationships with family and friends.[4]

Stress and other hazards have existed in offices for years. However, the trend towards computerisation is not only adding new problems and hazards but is also exacerbating the very job characteristics found to be stressful and eliminating those which promote job satisfaction and counteract stress. Recent research findings which show the high levels of stress experienced by clerical employees in "automated" offices have led to mounting concern over the impact of computerisation on the quality of working life and to strident calls for action to reduce stress at work.

The remainder of this chapter is broken down into three parts. The first section focuses on sources of stress for data-entry workers: these relate to some of the specific characteristics of the physical work environment, working time arrangements and work organisation which have been found critical with regard to both worker satisfaction and health. The second section discusses the role of individual differences in the stress syndrome. It includes some of the demographic, physiological and psychological characteristics of workers which are likely to influence their susceptibility and response to occupational stress. The third section focuses on the effects of occupational stress. These effects can be physiological, psychological or behavioural. They can take place in the short, medium or long term and can result in temporary or permanent maladaptive functioning or disability for the worker. In addition, occupational stress has repercussions for the worker's family, the organisation and the community.

SOURCES OF STRESS

The sources of stress for data-entry workers include work organisation and job content factors, working time, remuneration and incentive systems, and working environment factors. These conditions and job characteristics constitute the objective working environment of data-entry workers.

Just as these conditions and job characteristics overlap and interact, their effects on data-entry workers usually also result from a cumulative and combined set of job pressures and conditions. However, in this section we discuss only those aspects of data-entry jobs which have been empirically found to be particularly significant in inducing stress. This separation of sources of stress into various factors or categories is somewhat artificial and over-simplifies the dynamic interaction of different sources. None the less, it is useful to identify more specifically the sources of stress in order to take them into consideration when examining policies and strategies to improve data-entry jobs. This is particularly significant, since changes in all these factors can be expensive and disruptive and may, in some cases, be impossible. Therefore, it is important to isolate as far as possible the most powerful sources of occupational stress in order to concentrate on changes most likely to minimise or counteract their adverse effects.

Work organisation and job content factors

Particular properties and characteristics of data-entry jobs which relate to work organisation and job content are found to be critical sources of stress. They can conveniently be grouped into four main categories: quantitative overload, qualitative underload, lack of control over one's job and lack of social support.[5]

Quantitative overload

"Quantitative overload" means that one has too much to do in too little time. The main job characteristics which contribute to this problem include volume of work, task specialisation and standardisation, the need for close attention to detail, time pressure, work pace, certain forms of incentive systems and excessive supervision.

A number of factors can lead to an increased workload for data-entry workers. The computer's ability to process more information increases the demand for more data, on the assumption that more data result in more rational decision-making. This increase in demand is often not matched with a corresponding increase in the number of data-entry workers. The opposite is often the case: the introduction of new technology usually means a reduction in staff.

The application of factory-based time and motion studies and clerical work measurement schemes have been used to speed up work. For example, efficiency experts, using the queueing theory and work study techniques, have been able to increase the data-entry workload by 120 per cent.[6] In another case, an employee who had been eight years in a data-entry department describes the increased pressure to produce more where she works:

Everything seemed just fine at work until last summer, when a company-hired management consulting firm came to our department, supposedly to study how *management* could work better. But instead of improving management's operation, the consultant began to carefully measure and time *our* production speeds. We used to have to process a *maximum* of 4,000 checks a day. Now 4,000 has become the *minimum*—that's one check every 6 seconds—and the average they require is between 5,000 and 6,000— about 4 seconds per check.[7]

The extreme simplification and standardisation of tasks has also facilitated the introduction of piece-work and bonus systems to stimulate productivity. Incentive systems can be used to increase productivity and workload with relatively small increases in salaries. This is particularly true of work which is high in volume and low in complexity. An incentive system introduced in a huge American bank, for example, resulted in an 18.5 per cent increase in output with only a 6 per cent increase in the data-entry operator's salary. In this case, the operator was paid $40 per day for an output of 1,950 records. With the incentive system, if she entered an additional 1,700 records during a shift, she earned an additional $20. This meant a near-doubling of output for only a 50 per cent increase in salary.[8]

Supervisors can also exert pressure on the worker to increase her output. Indeed, some supervisors are under tremendous pressure themselves. In some cases, this pressure is aggravated by conflicting demands from various chiefs or "clients", who may all consider their work as priority and want it on a "rush" basis. The supervisor, aware that her job—or her promotion—partly depends on her responding to these demands, tends to transfer or counteract the pressure she is under by pushing the operators under her control to work faster and harder.

Certain practices, facilitated by the capabilities of modern hardware, also spur the data-entry operator to produce more. Modern hardware has allowed instant access to each worker's performance in terms of number of keystrokes, lines or pages entered. This has facilitated practices such as peer pressure or competition among workers. The posting of daily performance records, for example, "shames" the less productive workers while encouraging competition among the more productive. Sometimes, the operator receives direct feedback on performance via the terminal, which can lead to the constant feeling of being behind schedule.

In some cases, the increased productivity of the equipment and the operators has not been used to cut the volume of typing.[9] Instead, there has been an increase in the amount of retyping: authors are more likely to draft and redraft time and again or to send back documents for cosmetic changes (e.g. change headings from small letters to capitals). Moreover, the word-processing centre is sent every text and typing job regardless of its suitability for processing, including material which previously would not have been typed at all. These problems often result from a lack of knowledge on the part of users or "clients".

The design of the equipment itself can encourage the data-entry worker to work harder. This results from a "feeling" that the screen is "alive" and demands a response: the cursor is waiting to move to the next character position. The operator's activity is more continuous, particularly as the removal of paper handling and decision-making allows more time to input and encourages continuous working. The natural breaks in the tempo of work activity have been removed. This was shown, for example, in a study which compared the jobs of conventional copy typists and "video typists" in an engineering consultancy firm.[10] Moreover, since if the terminal was switched off, the video typist had to go through the "logging on" procedure to start again, it was found that she therefore stayed at the machine and was likely to work for longer periods than the copy typist without any change in activity.

An additional quantitative burden on the data-entry worker results from difficulties in accurately entering data contained in source documents and from corrections which must be made while work is being keyed. For example, operators can be required to work from source documents which are poorly handwritten or otherwise hard to read. Operators may also be expected, for example, to correct spelling or to check for likely errors (e.g. in bank cheques) while keying. Additional problems result when the source material is mostly meaningless coded data or highly technical matter such as chemical nomenclature. Often, the worker is not given extra time to compensate for these additional task demands. It is significant to note that these demands do not add up to variety and responsibility in data-entry work: they merely constitute an additional load on the worker.

Certain situations can exacerbate the stress that the operator already experiences from having too much to do in too little time. An additional source of stress which is often associated with quantitative overload is temporary machine breakdown and "slow" response time. For data-entry workers, a machine breakdown means an uneven workload because their work piles up while the system is out of action. These situations constitute an appreciable source of stress for data-entry workers. For example, an extensive study of female white-collar workers in an insurance company showed that the VDU operators (data-entry workers) felt more rushed, tense, frustrated and irritated while waiting for the system to start up again than during regular work.[11] To cope with such interruptions, a special strategy evolved: "the pace is forced early in the day to guard against any breakdown later on. This means that breakdowns affect the workload not only when they occur but even when they do not. The threat of breakdown is constantly present".[12] Consequently, the operator must enter as much text as she can as quickly as she can, in case the machine breaks down later on. It is interesting to note that this strategy of coping with the risk of stoppages is similar to that adopted in mechanised factory work where routines are largely dictated by the technology.[13] Computer breakdowns are not rare occurrences. In the above-mentioned insurance company study, unplanned interruptions usually occurred several times a week and the duration usually varied from a few minutes to several hours. The expected duration was usually announced, but not until at least 15 minutes after it had occurred.

System response time can also be a cause of stress. Prolongation of response times sometimes occurs as a result of the high load on the computer system. It is interesting to note that VDU operators in the above-mentioned insurance company preferred not to have to wait more than 5 seconds for the computer to respond.[14] When the previous "manual" system was used, it was quite acceptable for customers, management and employees to wait for several minutes; but the introduction of computers (and VDUs) had drastically increased the expectation for rapid information input and retrieval.[15] In the Symposium on Video Display Terminals and Vision of Workers, organised by the National Research Council in Washington, DC, one of the points raised was that "slow system response time and computer breakdowns can be especially frustrating and stressful, particularly in highly pressured work environments in which the workload is constant and heavy and in which production quotas are enforced".[16]

The period of introduction and adaptation of new data-entry equipment or systems can present particular problems concerning stress. During this phase, the operator is still learning the system, her speed or work pace is much slower and she is more likely to make mistakes. None the less, it may be the case that she is expected to attain a regular production quota. In such circumstances, she is very vulnerable to quantitative overload. This is especially true since the worker may be anxious about her ability to cope with the new technology.

Significant indicators of quantitative overload are recourse to overtime and inadequate or pre-empted rest pauses. Many data-entry operators cite frequent unexpected overtime, sometimes mandatory, to meet deadlines or handle seasonal heavy volumes of work.[17] Rest pauses can often be pre-empted as the worker attempts to meet production quotas and deadlines, particularly when the machine breaks down, when someone is away ill and her share is taken by the others, or when "clients" miss or ignore their own deadlines. Not only do these factors indicate quantitative overload, but they may also add to the stress already experienced by the data-entry worker as a result of her workload.

Quantitative overload was emphasised in a NIOSH study which compared the stress levels of clerical VDU operators, clerical non-VDU users and professionals using VDUs. The clerical VDU operators, compared with the two other groups, felt that the "workload was very heavy and that the work pace was too fast with little control over the pacing".[18] In a survey comparing subjective fatigue symptoms among 52 VDU operators (data-entry), 54 bank clerks and 66 city bus-drivers (control groups), the relationship between the workload and fatigue accumulation was highly significant for both VDU operators and city bus-drivers, but not for the bank clerks.[19]

Qualitative underload

"Qualitative underload" refers to impoverished job content. Such jobs are characterised by simple, repetitive tasks; little or no demand for creativity, problem-solving or full use of the worker's capabilities; almost no prospect for further learning and advancement; and limited scope for personal initiative and decision-making in determining work methods, work pace, and so on.

Numerous studies have shown that constrained routine jobs often lead to job dissatisfaction and instrumental attitudes to work (in other words, the degree to which work is valued primarily as a means to non-work ends rather than for its intrinsic rewards).[20] Moreover, there are also indications that such jobs, which "severely circumscribe autonomy, and the use of creative skills, come into conflict with basic human needs related to control, stimulus variation and self-expression and thus are detrimental to man both from a biological and social point of view".[21] Qualitative underload can be a powerful source of occupational stress.

It is important to understand that "the simplification of jobs and the absence of mental activity actually makes many jobs more demanding".[22] Jobs which call only for very limited skills but which place repeated demands on those skills are stressful in themselves. Early studies on the dysfunctional effects of industrial work revealed that fragmented, extremely specialised repetitive jobs led to problems of monotony and boredom. Such problems related to diminished alertness, decreased sensitivity to sensory input and, in some cases, to impaired muscular co-ordination.[23]

In data-entry jobs, many of the opportunities for decision-making and use of different skills have been taken over by the computer. For example, word processors relieve the operator of many of the aspects of typing which create some variety, such as document layout or format and presentation skills. The work pace and work sequence are also pre-determined. Although the capacities of the equipment may result in a decrease in physical exertion, this does not necessarily mean a cor-responding decrease in stress or mental tiredness. The contrary is often the case. Simplification and rigid standardisation have resulted in restricting the operator's job to the repetitive task of encoding.

Such specialisation means that mental demands are heavy but narrow. This limitation of activities to a small but demanding repertoire is a source of stress independent of quantitative workload (i.e. the volume of work). In fact, such a situation may be more likely to cause stress than monotonous physical work. This has been shown in several laboratory and field studies.[24] For example, studies by the USSR Academy of Sciences clearly point out that—

Occupational aspects of uniform monotonous mental work, generated by scientific and technical progress, render the problem more acute than does monotonous and variform physical work. The negative effects of such mental work are more profound than those of monotonous physical work.[25]

In addition, it is significant to note that assembly-line workers, for example, may find temporary relief from boredom by day-dreaming or chatting with fellow workers, for example. For data-entry workers, such momentary escape is often pre-empted by the need for close attention in entering data. Moreover, monitoring devices, prompters or cursors encourage the worker to concentrate on her work.

The lack of career opportunities also contributes to the degree of qualitative underload. Some of the problems related to careers were discussed in Chapter 2. Sometimes data-entry workers may hope that job evaluation will lead to an upgrading of their jobs. Unfortunately, in most cases, job evaluation schemes or grading systems may not have been revised to reflect the changes in the content of jobs resulting from computerisation by considering new approaches to certain factors or adjusting the weighting of existing factors in such schemes. For example, in Sweden weight is given to new factors introduced into job evaluation schemes, such as the extent of being tied to a work station, irregular work patterns and time pressure.[26] Since the design of the equipment absorbs some of the skills of the job, it may actually be the case that, under traditional job evaluation analysis, "the typists' job value and responsi-bilities will, at best, remain constant and not improve; at worst, they could go down and ultimately take the salary level expectations with them".[27]

For data-entry workers, the lack of career opportunities means that there is no escape in sight from the continuous daily stress resulting from the nature of the task. The lack of career opportunities therefore exacerbates the other sources of stress on the job.

Moreover, the introduction of word-processing equipment can be particularly stressful for older and more experienced workers. They suddenly find that, after years of service and experience, they could easily be replaced by a school-leaver with a few weeks of training. In fact, in terms of certain skill requirements (manual dexterity, close attention to detail, using the VDU) and in meeting production quotas, they may find themselves actually behind the young newcomers.

Other contributing factors to qualitative underload relate to certain characteristics of Taylorist organisation of work, such as: close supervision; lack of understanding of the overall job or work system as a result of job specialisation; inflexible routines and procedures; physical separation according to functions or tasks performed; and limited opportunities to learn and develop new skills on the job. For data-entry workers, it is these constraints to decision-making (and not decision-making *per se*) that cause stress.

Significantly, the constraints on decision-making and skill use facilitate the increase in the volume of work or quantitative overload. The fragmentation of the job and the use of the technology ensure that the worker concentrates solely on the repetitive task of encoding. This combination of too much work or high job demands (quantitative overload) which offer minimum interest, challenge and decision-making latitude (qualitative underload) is a particularly powerful source of stress for these low-status workers.[28] Some studies have shown that "the working individual with few opportunities to make decisions in the face of output pressure is most subject to job strain".[29]

Lack of control over one's job

All organisations have systems which control the distribution of work and regulate its quantity and quality. These control systems can, when taken to extremes, act as potent sources of occupational stress. In data-entry work, the following control system problems often act as sources of stress: computer-monitored work standards and performance; close supervision; over-rationalisation; and formalisation of the work process. In addition, computer breakdowns, prolonged system response time and delays in submission of texts by authors can contribute to the worker's feeling of lack of control over her job.

Many word-processing systems are designed to facilitate the enforcement of pre-established production quotas and speed of work. As previously mentioned, word-processing equipment can be programmed to measure key depressions automatically and to issue disciplinary warnings if input speeds and time at the machine do not meet management standards. In a study comparing clerical VDU users and clerical non-VDU users, the VDU users had higher levels of stress, although their job demands in terms of workload were the same as the non-users.[30] The difference in stress levels was attributed to the fact that the non-VDU users could set their own work pace during the day, while the VDU users—

... were monitored closely by the computer system which provided up-to-the-minute performance reports on the rate of production and error levels to supervisors. This produced a feeling in the clerical [VDU] operators that they were being constantly "watched" by the computer and controlled by the supervisors.[31]

They saw themselves in a highly controlled work environment that demanded high productivity. For these workers, the inflexible work system, which provided closer tracking over their performance, and the directive/corrective management style that it engendered, seemed to produce a feeling of loss of control over their work activity.

Moreover, the combination of continuous monitoring and constant automatic prompting often have the same effects as machine pacing in repetitive industrial work. Machine pacing has been found to be a source of stress in studies concerning, for example, assembly-line work. A similar type of monitoring is also used in keypunching jobs. In some keypunching departments, as mentioned in Chapter 2, each machine is wired to the supervisor's board which enables her to detect immediately if anyone stops punching. "There is no more efficient instrument of control from the top than machinery."[32]

The centralisation of data-entry work in word-processing pools or keypunch centres, and specialisation within the data-entry task, minimise, if they do not eliminate, opportunities for the worker to exercise control over her own work. The supervisor allocates the work to be keyed, the data-entry worker inputs the raw text according to set standards and specifications, and the proof-reader checks for errors. Moreover, close supervision—together with the failure or difficulty to understand the total work process and minimal contact with others, except with other data-entry workers and the supervisor—inhibits personal initiatives and control over the job.

Fragmented and specialised work requires inflexible routines to ensure that the subparts fit together. The introduction of computerisation also often leads to more rigid formalisation of the work process. More activities are programmed through the establishment and enforcement of procedures, rules and regulations and time control. In this connection, it is significant to note that data-entry workers are more subject to formal controls because their work has been reduced to standardised repetitive tasks.

Another factor which tends to increase the worker's feeling of lack of control over her work is the unpredictability of computer breakdowns. This is particularly critical for data-entry workers, who feel that their work rate and performance are dependent on the hardware. Consequently, when the computer breaks down, they see their work piling up but feel helpless to do anything about it. Moreover, since most data-entry workers do not have any secondary task to perform during these interruptions, they can only wait until the computer system starts functioning again.

A similar feeling occurs during prolonged response time. In such cases, the operator cannot tell whether the "silence" is due to computer breakdown, a higher load or her own error. This uncertainty adds to her burden, particularly when she has a large amount of work to encode.

Delay in incoming texts to be encoded can also contribute to the operator's feeling of lack of control over her job. This delay may be due to the "clients" not meeting their respective deadlines, or delays on the part of the supervisor, editor or proof-reader. Because the operator has no control over the work assigned to her, she finds the waiting periods stressful, indeed not very different from the effects of computer break-downs. This is particularly true since she knows that later on she will be rushed and overloaded.

Moreover, while a secretary can become angry with her chief for exercising strict control, a data-entry worker cannot easily target her resentment and frustration. She can only direct her anger towards her supervisor, while realising that the supervisor has no real power, or generally towards "them", the anonymous chiefs or "clients". This problem is compounded by grievance procedures which are described by some workers as "ineffective" or "arbitrary".[33]

Data-entry workers also experience ambiguity concerning their future job security. The formalisation of the work process, including detailed specification and standardisation of the elements of the task, the ambiguity of job classification systems and the perceived "arbitrariness" of grievance procedures make data-entry workers acutely aware that they are very expendable. Data-entry workers suffer from lack of control over their future on the job.

Finally, research studies have shown not only how the lack of control over one's own work can constitute a threat to health, but also how the worker's ability to counteract stress is generally better if she can exercise a reasonable degree of control over her work situation. One of these studies concluded that—

Under equal conditions with respect to loads and problems, the worker who can to some degree control the work situation in terms of work rhythm, sequences of operations and choice of methods is less subject to adverse effects than a worker who has to follow fully pre-structured sequences, cycles and methods.[34]

Lack of social support on the job

In Chapter 2, the constraints to significant and supportive relation-ships at work were described. These constraints relate to the nature of the task, the organisational control system and the organisational climate, especially the attitude of the immediate supervisor, office layout and personnel practices.

Relationships between interpersonal factors, illness and life expectancy have been studied both extensively and intensively. While these studies illustrate the role of a lack of social support as a source of stress, recent evidence also suggests that social support mitigates or buffers the effects of job-related stressful events on physical and mental health.[35] Several kinds of work-related stress are less marked for people with supportive relationships than for those who lack such support. These results have held, with significant but imperfect consistency, in a variety of settings and research designs, including studies on overload in administrative jobs and monotonous work.

Supportive relationships can modify or buffer potentially negative effects of stress either by reducing the stress itself or by facilitating the worker's efforts to deal with it. Supportive fellow-workers are less likely to create interpersonal conflicts and tensions. For example, because of peer support and group cohesiveness, workers may share or distribute work among themselves or assist a particular worker in such cases as heavy workload or "covering" during breaks or periods of informal leave. Supervisors can foster collaboration, instead of competition, among the data-entry workers. Supportive fellow-workers may facilitate dealing with and adaptation to stress by showing concern and making the person feel positively about herself and her job; by conveying a sense of belonging; or by providing tangible help when needed and suggesting ways of coping with the situation.

In spite of its buffering effect, social support should not be considered as a substitute for efforts to reduce the incidence of occupational stress at the workplace. Although social support may be rewarding in many ways, work enterprises should not expect supervisors and fellow workers, much less spouses, friends and relatives of fellow workers to buffer employees against stresses which the organisation can reasonably reduce or prevent entirely.[36]

Interaction of work organisation and job content factors

As is evident from the above discussion, the sources of stress relating to work organisation and job content interact. This interaction results in part from the structural interdependence of organisational characteristics. The organisational characteristics which are of particular relevance to data-entry workers are centralisation and specialisation, formalised means of monitoring and control, and hierarchies of authority. When word processing or other forms of data entry are introduced, an organisational decision is often made to take advantage of centralisation and specialisation in order to achieve productivity benefits. Simultaneously, the application of time and motion concepts results in fragmented, standardised jobs and the concentration of machines on a functional basis. The workers are subjected to stringent controls and formal rules in order to assure that productivity gains are maintained. These data-entry centres are related to the document cycle through external hierarchical control.

Thus, there is a "package" of organisational characteristics which tends to accompany the setting up of a data-entry workplace. It is therefore usual to find all the above sources of stress present at the same time in data-entry or word-processing centres.

Several studies have demonstrated how sources of stress to do with work organisation interact in the specific case of data-entry work.

A field investigation of health complaints and job stress in video display operations was carried out by NIOSH in five different work sites.[37] Clerical VDU operators reported significantly higher levels of job stress and fatigue than professionals using VDUs and a control group of clerical non-VDU users. This high level of stress was associated with increased workload, greater work pressure and supervision, lack of control over job activities, boredom, uncertainty about job future and lower self-esteem experienced by the clerical VDU operators as compared with the two other groups. The results of this study indicate that the degree of stress and health problems experienced by the three groups were linked to the nature or type of jobs they performed—

When the job features of the various groups are examined we see that the clerical VDT [= VDU] operators held jobs involving rigid work procedures with high production standards, constant pressure for performance, very little operator control over job tasks, and little identification with and satisfaction from the end-product of their work activity. In contrast to the clerical VDT operators, the professionals using VDTs held jobs that allowed for flexibility, control over job tasks, utilisation of their education and a great deal of satisfaction and pride in their end-product. While both jobs had tight deadline requirements, the professional operators had a great deal of control over how these would be met. In their case, the VDT was a tool that could be used for enhancing their end-product, while for the clerical VDT operators, the VDT was part of a new technology that took more and more meaning out of their work. It's not surprising that the professionals using VDTs did not report levels of job stress as high as the clerical VDT operators. . . . This suggests that the use of the VDT is not the only factor contributing to operator stress levels and health complaints, but that job content also makes a contribution.[38]

A study in an insurance company of the importance of job content for workers who spent more than 50 per cent of their time working with VDUs was undertaken by the Department of Psychology of the University of Stockholm as part of a bigger study on stress in computerised administrative work.[39] Workers were grouped according to how they used or interacted with the computer. One group consisted of personnel from the customer service section, who used the computer to feed in or to retrieve information on the basis of customer contacts by phone or in person; the other group ("data-entry") consisted of employees from various departments whose main task was to feed in ("code") data to the computer system on the basis of incoming documents.

The effects of the changes in job content after computerisation were mainly negative for both groups, although this tendency was more pronounced for the data-entry group. Both groups also reported that the number of routine tasks and the demand for attention and concentration had increased. However, the data-entry group, unlike the customer service group, considered that the work now had less variety. Autonomy in planning and executing daily tasks had decreased for both groups, but the tendency was more pronounced for the data-entry group. No member of either group, however, considered that the demand for attention, mental strain or number of routine tasks had decreased since the introduction of VDUs.[40]

It is interesting to note that one of the main findings of the overall study was that the mental strain in VDU work was determined to a large extent by the nature of the tasks.[41] In general, workers whose jobs involved dealing with customers for settling claims and calculating tariffs, and who spent less than half of their working hours at VDUs, reported fewer problems with the computer system. They considered the VDU as just another aid which enabled them to obtain a complete picture of an insurance case. They also had a higher degree of personal control over the amount of work that they did, and its pace. Most of their stress problems had to do with their perception of heavy responsibility at work. Their common health complaint was stomach problems. On the other hand, workers carrying out extensive VDU work experienced greater mental strain because of the workload, high demands on concentration, uncertainty of computer breakdown and lack of control over their work, which were confirmed by physiological measurements of catecholamine excretion, heart rate and blood pressure. They also suffered from complaints concerning pains in the arms, neck, shoulders and back, headaches and eye fatigue. Workers who fared worst were those whose main task was to feed the computer system with current data from documents.[42]

A similar study concerned female VDU operators who carried out two different types of VDU tasks.[43] One task consisted of data acquisition in banks, where the computer was used solely for data input. The other task involved a dialogue with the computer in a publishing house and a pharmaceutical firm. The results of the study were interpreted in the light of task content. Data acquisition was a fragmented task characterised by frequent visual sweeps between the VDU and the documents, limited decision-making, low knowledge and skill requirements, and very short cycle times. In comparison, dialogue required some routine decisions and was characterised by higher knowledge and skill requirements and longer work cycles.

Not surprisingly, the data acquisition group had a higher frequency of psychosomatic disorders, nervous disturbances and inadequate sleep patterns. One of the conclusions of the study was that "simple, repetitive work, lacking interest and full use of the operator's capabilities, and its psychosocial consequences explain in large part the job dissatisfaction expressed by the majority of operators".[44]

A survey of 2,330 workers in 15 workplaces was conducted by the Labour Education and Studies Centre of the Canadian Labour Congress (now CLC-Educational Services) in order to examine the nature and extent of health-related problems among office workers.[45] It compared the responses of VDU and non-VDU users. The jobs of respondents were classified into four main types of work, as follows:

(a) production-line jobs (e.g. telephone operators and reservation agents);

(b) data-entry jobs (e.g. word-processing operators and typists);

(c) "conversational clerical jobs" (e.g. clerks using VDUs for information storage and retrieval and general office clerical staff); and

(d) professional and technical jobs (e.g. computer programmers and television production workers using VDUs and professional and administrative personnel not using VDUs).[46]

Overall, workers whose jobs required intensive use of VDUs (especially in categories (a) and (b)) reported significantly more types of and more severe health problems, as well as higher levels of stress.[47] These intensive VDU users also reported less control over the speed of their work, greater work pressure and limited opportunities to perform non-VDU tasks.[48]

Working time

Three working-time issues are particularly relevant to stress. These are overtime, rest pauses and shift work.

As previously mentioned, frequent recourse to overtime is encouraged by the heavy volume of work, particularly in the event of machine breakdowns, failure of "clients" to meet their respective deadlines, staff cut-backs and absences of fellow workers, and in order to meet seasonal demands or deadlines. In some countries, the development and initial start-up of new data-processing systems have reportedly led to a "situation of chronic overtime and intensified mental stress for operators . . . ".[49] In some cases, overtime is mandatory, while in others, although not obligatory, it is expected. As one worker in a magazine company said: "It's not absolutely mandatory to accept overtime, but 'flexibility' is one of the qualities you are rated for".[50]

Overtime extends the performance of an already stressful job and reduces the time or possibilities for rest and recovery after work. Since data-entry jobs are often characterised by increased workload and work intensity (i.e. by physical and mental stress), prolonging the daily working hours means prolonging the workers' exposure to stress. Moreover, the overtime load often calls for intense adaptive efforts, the effects of which are not only restricted to the extra hours worked but also "carried over" to affect the time spent in leisure, family or other personal activities.

The importance of rest pauses to counteract or minimise the negative effects of fatigue and stress was discussed in Chapter 2. However, rest pauses are also important from another perspective. Firstly, they should not themselves be a source of stress. For example, fixed rest pauses may mean that the data-entry worker cannot take a break when she needs it, or the pause may be so regimented that it exacerbates the worker's feeling of being "treated like a child" and the lack of control over her job. In such circumstances, the provision of the rest pause undermines its very purpose. Secondly, to the extent possible, workers should be given some leeway in deciding when to take their rest pauses. However, such variable rest pause frequency should not lead to delay or omission because of the heavy volume of work. Thirdly, the level of fatigue and stress experienced by the worker, and thus the timing of rest pauses, should not be based on some measure of work efficiency (i.e. performance or productivity) alone. Performance or productivity measures may be misleading because when people realise that they are getting tired they tend to compensate by increased will-power or effort to carry on with the job, which in some cases leads to increased productivity or output.

An additional source of stress linked to working time is shift work. However, the extent of shift work among data-entry workers is evolving, and it remains to be seen whether shift work will become common with the development and wider application of word-processing and other office technologies. Where shift work, particularly night work, exists, studies have shown that it may be associated with health problems and difficulties in family and social life.

Remuneration and incentive systems

There are two main issues concerning the relationship of stress to pay. The first of these relates to the effect of deskilling and narrowed responsibilities on the level of pay, in particular the possibilities for pay reduction. The second concerns the possibilities certain incentive systems have for augmenting the work pace and undermining opportunities for co-operation and social support on the job.

Data-entry jobs, as previously described, are characterised by low-level, narrow skill requirements, limited scope for decision-making and overall lack of complexity. It is, therefore, not surprising that the introduction of word-processing technologies could lead to jobs which are downgraded and with reduced pay. Traditional job evaluation schemes usually emphasise job characteristics which are particularly lacking or weak in data-entry jobs. Consequently, the reduction in pay as a result of reclassification of the job could be an additional source of stress. For example, the Office Worker Health and Safety survey conducted in the United States by the Working Women Education Fund showed that the majority of the participating clerical workers ranked "low pay" as the second in their list of sources of occupational stress.[51]

Payment by results can often exacerbate other sources of stress on the job. However, it must be admitted at the outset that it is difficult to isolate the effects of a remuneration system from other factors which affect the worker's perception and behaviour at a particular point in time. For example, it is evident that work organisation, job content and remuneration system are closely linked. Specifically, in order to apply payment by results, particularly a piece-rate system, the tasks or operations carried out by the worker must be measurable. As a rule, this implies a rather narrow and repetitive job.[52]

Several studies on industrial work have shown that payment by results tends to lead to increased work pace, greater risk-taking, dysfunctional competition between individuals or teams, and higher accident rates.[53]

For data-entry jobs, payment by results can now be applied easily. Time and motion studies and work measurement techniques have made possible the setting of output standards. Individual performance can automatically be monitored and compared with the standard. Payment by results can be applied on the basis of the number of keystrokes, the number of records or other data keyed or the amount of time to input a specific quantity of raw text.

As previously mentioned, payment by results is a significant contributing factor to quantitative overload in so far as it is one of the main mechanisms used to " motivate" the worker to produce more. Since the physical effort she exerts is directly related to the cash payment she will receive, she is encouraged to work at a faster pace and more intensely. Payment by results could easily be instrumental in raising work intensity to harmful levels. This is particularly true if one considers the possibilities for "rate-cutting" inherent in some payment-by-results incentive schemes. Once the productivity standard for each incentive level is reached by most of the workers, it may be raised, forcing the data-entry worker to work harder to achieve the same incentive rate. It is hardly surprising that, in some cases, data-entry workers perceive payment-by-results schemes as a "ruse" designed to ensure the survival of the fittest.

Payment by results, particularly piece-rates, can also aggravate the worker's feeling that she is losing control over her job and that the computer is taking over. For example, a study of 50 VDU input typists performing piecework and 130 VDU input typists doing the same kind of work, but not on piecework, showed that the changes in factors such as sociability, frame of mind, state of stress, fatigue and inner security were much greater for those doing piecework.[54] VDU operators had strong feelings that "their work is the subject of control if the job is of a more routine nature, e.g. data entry, and all the more so if they are performing piecework".[55]

Payment by results may also lead to unpleasant jealousies and competition which undermine co-operation and group cohesion. Individuals under payment-by-results systems are likely to be less disposed to help each other, while group payment by results can place heavy social pressure on individual workers and sometimes leads to the expulsion of members who do not meet performance expectations. These effects can be exacerbated by public posting of individual or group performance and by contests or other techniques which encourage comparison and competition.

Working environment factors

In Chapter 3, the increasing importance of occupational health, safety and ergonomics with respect to data-entry work was discussed. Some of the factors relating to equipment design and workplace layout were examined, particularly those which warrant careful consideration.

Rigorous research has been undertaken to investigate the linkages between working environment factors and their immediate medical or physiological consequences. Most of the research findings concerning eye-strain, headaches, back pains, etc., suffered by data-entry workers relate these problems to the physical aspects of VDU use. This realisation has led to working environment standards and guide-lines in many areas such as lighting, noise, ergonomic design of visual screens, keyboards and chairs.

However, it is more difficult to investigate the linkages between stress and these physical working environment and equipment design factors. There is a tendency to conduct separate analyses of such factors and of the aspects of tasks relating to work content sources of stress, as previously discussed. In most research, working environment factors are usually considered under the headings of "physiological", "medical", "ergonomic" or "safety and health" aspects of VDU use, while other factors concerning work organisation and job content, remuneration and working-time arrangements fall under the headings of "psychosocial", "psychological" or "social" aspects. Such a dichotomy obviously entails different frames of reference, methodologies, instruments, hypotheses and assumptions.[56] In spite of this dichotomy, the physiological and psychological causes and effects of stress are inter-related, a fact which results in frequent references in one type of study to ideas relevant to the other. In the following section, the interaction between working environment and work organisation factors are examined.

Interaction between working environment and work organisation factors

In analysing the stress experienced by data-entry VDU operators, the contributions of work, equipment and workplace design factors must be considered. Stress in extensive VDU use often results from the interaction of physical design characteristics of the equipment and working environment, and organisational and job content variables. These different elements interact to either amplify or attenuate occupational stress.

In the previously mentioned NIOSH study which compared professional VDU users, clerical non-VDU users and clerical VDU operators, clerical VDU operators reported the highest levels of job stress and health complaints.[57] One of the main conclusions drawn from this investigation is that "a number of interacting factors including job task related features (job content, task requirements, workload) and environmental factors (lighting, work station design) contributed to the observed levels of job stress and health complaints".[58]

The study which compared the work and symptoms of two groups of female VDU operators—the data acquision and dialogue groups—also showed the interaction between the physical working environment and job content factors.[59] It is recalled that the data acquisition group's main task was limited to data input, while the dialogue group's job included searching for information, posing questions to the computer and interpreting responses. Recordings of eye movements were used to evaluate the length of uninterrupted looks and the frequency of visual sweeps (i.e. displacement of look from the visual display to documents or the keyboard) for each of the two groups. The results of the study show that, for the data acquisition group, the length of uninterrupted look is significantly shorter and the frequency of sweeping glances much higher than for the dialogue group.

These differences correspond to the different levels of information processing for the two groups. The shorter duration of uninterrupted looks and the higher frequency of visual sweeps between visual display and documents are determined by a fragmented task with a poor cognitive content. They are consistent with the job characteristics of data acquisition operators, which may be summed up as limited decision-making, less necessary learning, a lower degree of freedom and short cycle times. The psychosocial consequences of such simple, repetitive work are reflected in the job dissatisfaction experienced by the majority of the data acquisition operators (70 per cent compared with 28 per cent of the dialogue group), as well as in their significantly higher frequency of psychosomatic disorders, nervous disturbances and inadequate sleep patterns.

A significantly larger number of data acquisition operators reported symptoms of visual strain (glare discomfort, headaches, prickly sensation, blurred vision and visual acuity) and body pains (neck, right shoulder, upper and lower back). The visual strain experienced by the operators is related to the lighting of the workplace and the visual exploration characteristics of the task. This is exacerbated in data acquisition offices by the large windows which let in too much light and by the increased frequency of visual sweeps between the visual display and the documents, which have different luminances. Similarly, posture problems, which are more pervasive among the data acquisition group, are related to the characteristics of the job, particularly the lower degree of freedom, the piece-rate system and long periods of work in a seated position. The researchers emphasise that symptoms of visual strain and body pain must be examined from a holistic point of view, taking into account the operator and the job.

In spite of the extensive literature on occupational stress, little research has been done on the interaction of these two sets of potential sources of stress. Such integrated studies are necessary as a result of the pervasive changes in working environment and work content associated with VDU use. Failure to consider organisational aspects of VDU work (e.g. worker discretion, skill use and social support) together with working environment factors (e.g. VDU and work station design, and ambient environmental conditions) may result in distorted or limited findings concerning the stressful effects of VDU use and measures for their control.

The open-plan office

A major aspect of the working environment which may interact with other sources of stress, such as other environmental factors or work content factors, is the physical layout of the office. Some of these interactions were briefly mentioned in Chapters 2 and 3. However, to highlight the way in which the various sources of stress interact, we consider here the problems that may arise in the increasingly popular open-plan office, sometimes known as the "open" or "open landscape design" office. This type of office layout is frequently used for data-entry work.

There are many variations of the open-plan office. However, it is generally characterised by the absence of fixed interior walls and rooms, which in conventional offices define private work spaces. Instead, either totally open work areas or free-standing partitions and movable screens may be used to separate a particular work area or work station.

Private conventional offices are being replaced more and more by open-plan offices, primarily for economic reasons.[60] For new office construction, the building costs of open-plan offices are lower and the system is said to release more space. Moreover, the open-plan office also allows organisations to change or remodel the office layout more cheaply and quickly. This high degree of flexibility may be extremely important to accommodate both the introduction of new technologies, such as word processing and electronic mail, and changes in staffing requirements. Tax advantages, at least in the United States, are another consideration: fixed wall partitions must be depreciated over many years as part of the building, while open-plan office partitions can be depreciated in a much shorter time as office equipment. Another advantage cited by proponents of this concept is improved worker efficiency. This may result from better communication and more efficient routing and work flow. Finally, it is claimed that the system places greater emphasis on making the office a pleasant and attractive place to work. Most companies add colour and variety by using plants and pictures in the open-plan office.

However, not everyone is thoroughly convinced of the merits of the open-plan office. Many employees indicate that they experience the new open space as a "fish bowl", "cage", "warehouse", "bull pen" or "rat maze".[61] This less than enthusiastic response on the part of workers suggests that the physical layout of the open-plan office could contribute to stress.

As previously mentioned, although VDUs are less noisy than conventional typewriters, they are rarely completely silent. Moreover, the frequency may be annoying to some people with sensitivity to high-frequency noise and to those whose task requires close concentration. The problem is compounded when several VDUs are located close to each other in the same room. In some cases, the situation is also aggravated if printers or telecopiers are in the same work area and if acoustic hoods, screens or other sound-absorbing materials are inadequate.

Other types of noise-related distractions are also exacerbated in the open-plan office. People talking and telephones buzzing or ringing can be particularly irritating. In some cases, the auditory feedback—bleep, buzzer or click—incorporated in the VDU, which aids the operator to detect omitted and duplicate keystrokes, can disturb the concentration of the operators. In an open-plan office where there are a number of VDUs side by side, when the sound is heard each data-entry operator looks for a mistake on her screen.[62] Not only does this interrupt concentration and give rise to moments of anxiety, but it often also leads to the operator increasing the volume of her buzzer, click or bleep to ensure that she knows when it is she who made the mistake.

Many employees feel that they do not have enough privacy in an open-plan office.[63] In some open-plan office arrangements, they resent the notion of being constantly within sight and sound of the supervisor. As previously mentioned, line-of-sight geography (one of the characteristics of the open-plan office layout) allows visual observation of various work centres from a distant site, usually from the supervisor's location. This awareness of being under constant scrutiny both affects the workers' concentration on the job and prevents significant social interaction. It represents a considerable constraint to individual freedom and, by limiting opportunities for isolation and privacy, it also reduces the possibility of developing close interpersonal relationships. Many workers also report that, contrary to one of its purposes, it may undermine co-operation and community spirit.

In another study, the reactions of workers to a change from conventional to open-plan offices were examined with particularly careful control. Not only were there no changes in technology, duties or salary, but a control group was used to ensure that the attitudes measured related to open-plan offices and not to other factors. The conclusion reached was as follows:

Results of this study provide substantial support for the proposition that the physical context of an organisation has important implications for the quality of employees' work experiences. In particular, results showed that employees' internal motivation and satisfaction with work and colleagues declined sharply after moving from a conventional, multi-cellular office to an open-plan office containing no walls or partitions. . . . These results suggest that the physical space itself, rather than other extraneous factors, was responsible for the changes that occurred in the experimental group.[64]

Moreover, it is apparent that conditions under which open-plan offices have negative or positive consequences for the worker depend to a large extent on the nature of the task. For example, in the Swedish study comparing customer service and data-entry groups, the open-plan office had more negative consequences (e.g. "lack of peace and seclusion") for the data-entry group.[65]

THE ROLE OF INDIVIDUAL DIFFERENCES

As is evident from the previous section, there are many potentially stressful circumstances (sources of stress) within the data-entry workplace. Some are predominantly "objective" and quantifiable (e.g. quantitative overload, glare), and some rather more qualitative (e.g. lack of social support). However, not all workers will experience a given job situation as stressful; individuals react differently to the same (objective) situation. Neither will a given worker experience all job situations as equally stressful; the same individual may react differently to two situations presumed equally stressful. Moreover, even if several workers report the same amount of stress in their work, they may not necessarily incur the same type or degree of psychological or physiological response or, ultimately, illness. Individual differences have an important role in the experience of or response to work stress.

Given the extent and complexity of human variability, individual differences are one of the most complicated and difficult issues in stress research. None the less, most of the prevailing models of the stress syndrome, in spite of the existing semantic confusion and differences in perspective, view stress not as something cxogenous, but as a product of the dynamic mismatch between the individual and his or her physical or social environment. This interactive approach to stress holds that it is the combination of the particular situation and a given individual with his or her specific personal characteristics, expectations, past experience, aptitudes, attitudes and life circumstances that may result in a stress-inducing imbalance. Stress is likely to occur when there is a poor fit between the individual and his or her environment. It therefore becomes crucial to consider what characteristics of the individual influence the response to potential sources of occupational stress.

In discussing workers' characteristics, two points should be kept in mind. First, these characteristics can vary over time for each individual worker. For example, as workers grow older they modify their needs and expectations. This volatility of workers' characteristics can have important implications for the severity of the stress and for the multiplicity of stresses experienced by the individual at a particular point in time. Moreover, the particular state (physical and/or psychological) of the worker at the time the stress is imposed may also be a critical factor. In addition, each specific characteristic can be interpreted both positively or negatively, that is as a resource or as a limitation (or constraint). For example, skills and qualifications can be a resource in meeting the requirements of the job or a constraint if the job is simple and the worker is unchallenged or bored by it.

Workers vary on a whole range of dimensions and characteristics, some of which are more obvious and more objectively measurable than others. These include age, sex, marital status and socio-economic situation, skills and qualifications. Other dimensions such as personality, work attitudes and expectations are more qualitative in nature. Obviously, all these characteristics interact and influence the stress experienced by the worker on and off the job.

Age

Most workers increase their general knowledge about their jobs with age. When performance is determined by intellectual capacity, it is little affected by age. This is true of many occupations, including most of those of a clerical nature. However, for data-entry work, the task requirements place emphasis on motor and visual skills, which have been shown to frequently decline with age. Early research in gerontology dealing with sensory and motor abilities has consistently indicated that a decline does occur with age. This was found to be true of speed of movement, dexterity and co-ordination, physical strength, visual and auditory sensitivity and perceptual speed.

For example, age has profound effects on the ability of the eye to "sharp-focus" objects at varying distances (power of accommodation) because the lens gradually loses its elasticity. The performance-related task requirements of data-entry work may be more analogous to those in factory jobs, where workers are more vulnerable to the effects of ageing. Although older factory workers typically can perform various duties as well as those who are much younger, they cannot repeat the operations over and over again at the same rate or pace. To the extent that older workers have full-time data-entry jobs, they would be expected to have to work harder to attain the same performance level as younger workers. In view of the requirements of the job, therefore, it is not surprising that a number of job descriptions for data-entry work specify young workers.

Sex, marital status and socio-economic situation

The main characteristics of data-entry workers in terms of sex, marital status and socio-economic situation can be summarised as follows:

(1) Almost all data-entry workers are women.

(2) Many, if not most, of these women are married, and the proportion of married women is increasing; there is a significant growing number of data-entry workers who are single parents or heads of households.

(3) Pay is relatively low, in many cases below the poverty level, especially for single parents.

(4) Such single parents tend to be overburdened with responsibilities, insecurity and scarce resources.

(5) Educational levels are approximately the same as for workers in general.

There seems to be little doubt of the relationship between stress and the work/family interface. The effects of stress can be influenced by individual differences relating to family roles. However, this important area has been relatively neglected in stress research—

Most models or frameworks for the study of occupational stress . . . tack on a panel of variables usually termed "extra-organisational", to capture the influence of family or life stress on the already occupationally stressed individual. Unfortunately, this panel of variables is almost never examined. Each life domain has been treated as a closed system and the interaction between work and family has been largely ignored.[66]

The entry of women into the paid workforce meant largely the expansion of demands on them. This is particularly true for economically active women with dependent children, who now assume the demanding multiple roles of wife, mother and worker. Each of these roles involves several activities which are supposed to be performed by a single person, with the result that the person is likely to experience stress caused by role conflict and role overload. Role conflict or overload occur when two or more demands are made on the person at the same time, such that compliance with one would make compliance with the other more difficult. Conflict or overload can be generated by two competing demands of two roles held by the same person. For example, the role of the worker may require the employed woman to do overtime, while her role as a mother may require her to attend a school function. Some researchers have suggested that women who are engaged in paid work and who have a family have two *simultaneous* roles, whereas men in the same position tend to have *sequential* roles.[67] Men's family responsibilities often tend to be handled during the evening after work, while women's family responsibilities continue throughout the day.

Irrespective of the stress-induced demands of multiple roles, women who are economically active have a greater workload. Studies of the weekly round of such women indicate a range of averages of 50–80 hours a week in housework, child-care and paid labour. Although men are beginning to share some of these family-related tasks, "when a woman with a child takes a job today, she is typically adding her work week to a 30- to 40-hour 'home-making' minimum . . .".[68]

Obviously, the above-mentioned problems are exacerbated for single-parent working mothers. Their plight is more dismal because of their economic situation and their limited opportunity to improve their earning power. The few studies on work and family, which have tended to focus on women in managerial or professional positions, are often interpreted as representative of working women. Although there may be similarities between a female lawyer and a data-entry worker, the differences are usually more important. In particular, the data-entry worker, because of her lower income, almost always has greater difficulties in fulfilling family responsibilities, especially if she is a single parent.

Skills and qualifications

One of the most important determinants of how a worker reacts to a job is the level of skill and qualifications that she has in order to perform it. When a worker does not have the required aptitude, skill or qualifications to perform the job, serious problems develop for both the worker and the organisation. For the organisation, underskilled or underqualified workers generate numerous direct and indirect costs, such as low output, poor-quality work, extra supervisory time, etc. For the worker, being underskilled and underqualified can cause considerable anxiety and embarrassment.

Variations in aptitude and skill modify the extent to which sources of stress impinge upon the worker, particularly quantitative overload and qualitative underload. Aptitudes refer to discrete traits or abilities which are indicative of the capacity to gain proficiency or to learn. They indicate potential for certain kinds of work, and can be developed into skills through training. Skills refer to proficiency in performing a particular task.

For data-entry work, specific clerical aptitudes and skills are required. These clerical aptitudes include speed and accuracy in perceiving numerical and verbal similarities and differences, verbal skill (spelling, vocabulary, reading comprehension), numerical skill (error location, arithmetical computation), fine manual dexterity, and so on. With training and experience, skill in keypunching or typing are developed. A data-entry worker's level of skill, particularly typing or keying, is a significant factor in influencing her ability to cope with the volume of work (quantitative overload). For the inexperienced data-entry operator, movements are more complex and uncertain, and therefore slower. A large proportion of her time and effort is concerned with aspects of how to do the task, such as learning and exploring, rather than dealing directly with the demands of the task. In this case, it would be expected that the worker would have greater difficulty in meeting the output requirements of the job and would thus experience a quantitative overload.

The qualifications of the data-entry worker can also influence the way in which she reacts to her job. Unlike the situation with respect to aptitudes and skills, data-entry workers are often overqualified in terms of their general education and possibly their experience. Overqualified data-entry workers are likely to find themselves unchallenged, frustrated and bored by the job. For these workers, the stress effects of qualitative underload can be exacerbated.

In some cases, selection, including testing, may increase or diminish congruence between the worker and the job. On the one hand, numerous tests and models for selection and placement are used in matching people to jobs so that all workers have the capability to perform adequately. On the other, since those candidates who score highest on the tests are routinely selected, a frequent side-effect of the "test-selection" approach is that many workers turn out to be overqualified for the job they are to do.

Personality and work attitudes

According to Ghiselli and Brown—

Success on a job is not solely determined by ability but is also attributable in part to traits of personality, character and interest. . . . Personality refers to those traits of the individual or those aspects of his behavior that have emotional, social, motivational or moral connotations. . . . [69]

However, it must be recognised that the concept of personality, like the stress syndrome, is difficult to define, with each school of thought analysing it from its own unique perspective. None the less, there seem to be certain commonalities in conceptualising personality. Personality is not a thing or tangible object to be defined and identified; rather it is an inference of abstraction that calls to mind the individuality, adaptability and characteristic dispositions of the human organism. Although personality is largely a differentiating concept, there are certain dimensions and facets that are present in everyone.

Personality attributes and personal experience can influence or "condition" the way in which workers perceive and respond to stress at work.

Perhaps the most widely discussed personality characteristic with respect to occupational stress is the Type A and Type B differentiation described by two American cardiologists, Friedman and Rosenman.[70] They found that individuals whom they referred to as Type A were a much higher coronary risk than those whom they called Type B. Type A personality is characterised by intense striving for achievement, competitiveness, easily provoked impatience, time urgency, abruptness of gesture and speech, over-commitment to vocation or profession, and excessive drive and hostility. Type B, the exact antithesis or converse of Type A, is characterised by an easy-going behaviour pattern. However, it is difficult to know to what extent the Type A behaviour is a risk factor across different occupational and work settings. The basic evidence comes from a male sample which is only 10 per cent blue collar, with most of the remainder from middle and upper levels of managerial and technical-scientific work. Moreover, there are studies which contradict the generalisation that managers are more prone to coronary heart disease and that they are necessarily Type A individuals.[71] While this area of research increases knowledge concerning managerial or executive stress, it is still not clear to what extent such personality profiles are applicable to female managers, let alone to female clerical workers.

There are several personality variables that have been shown to facilitate understanding of some of the variations in thought and behaviour that differentiate one person from another. Although some of these variables have been included in job satisfaction studies, their specific relationships to stress still remain to be investigated. None the less, they are briefly described here because they seem at least intuitively related and could perhaps account for part of the differences in perception and experience of stress.

Some researchers have found that certain individuals tend to be more categorical and more disposed to moral judgements in their reactions to others, intellectually rigid, hostile in response to restraints, deferential to those above and exploitative of those below, and fearful of social change. Some studies have shown that these personality characteristics can partly differentiate persons who work more productively under "democratic" leaders and those who produce more under close directive supervision.[72] The degree to which this personality dimension is characteristic of some data-entry workers may influence in part their reactions to various sources of stress on the job concerning the type of supervision, the implications of change to computerisation and social interaction among fellow workers.

Other researchers have differentiated human personalities according to their degree of conformity versus independence of judgement.[73] Simply, some individuals are more likely to yield to group pressure or consensus than others. The relatively more independent-minded individuals are likely to be more creative, to value originality of ideas and to prefer change and variety to routine and certainty, and do not particularly admire stringent self-discipline and tireless devotion to duty. It is likely that, for the more "independent" data-entry workers, the highly structured workplace, the routine repetitive nature of the data-entry task and the need to exert extra effort (overtime, increased workload, etc.) may be powerful sources of stress.

Another personality factor on which much research has been carried out relates to ambition, accomplishment, achievement and prestige.[74] For success-oriented data-entry workers, the dearth of career opportunities, the lack of recognition and the lack of a sense of completion of a whole and indentifiable piece of work can influence their perception and level of stress. These data-entry workers may also find working in a pool particularly stressful, since they may perceive their individual contribution as lost in the larger setting. The lack of overall control over one's work is also likely to be perceived as a potent source of stress.

In a similar vein, researchers have looked at individual differences in terms of the need for affiliation.[75] Individuals with strong social needs might find the lack of opportunities for significant social relationships in data-entry jobs particularly stressful.

Some researchers have looked at the differences in orientation of workers in terms of their job and non-job interests.[76] Similar to role conflict, data-entry workers may find that meeting the demands both of their job and of outside activities is a source of stress. Moreover, data-entry workers who are more job oriented may find that the jobs they hold do not meet their expectations.

Thus far, we have discussed how some individual differences moderate or influence the stress experienced by data-entry workers. The worker's age, sex, marital status, socio-economic position, skills, qualifications, and personality and work attitudes can influence when and to what extent certain situations or events are stressful for a particular individual. It was emphasised that some of these individual characteristics vary over time, due in part to experience both on and off the job, and in part to personal growth.

In spite of the significance of individual differences in moderating stress, it is important not to treat stress problems solely at the level of the individual. This approach "tends to convert problems in the work environment to private problems. Also, the pressure to adapt is directed toward the individual and not toward the organisation and the production process".[77] While most formulations of stress concern the use of subjective approaches, this does not mean that stress problems necessarily have personal causes or should be treated solely as "personal" problems. The fact that stress has a cognitive component or that individual differences can modify the perception, tolerance and severity of stress does not mean that the sources of stress discussed at the beginning of this chapter are not real or objective.

There is likely to be some discrepancy between objective conditions at work and each individual's perception. Various mental mechanisms, such as defences, can distort a person's perception. In fact, a worker may simply "not know what is right or useful for him with regard to the defined tolerable conditions of health and well-being . . .".[78] Workers do not have a self-regulating internal mechanism that will guarantee that they will take action before being harmed. For example, they may ignore their own need for rest pauses or work on the VDU all day to cope with the workload. Workers may not be aware of the long-term impact of work stress; they may not realise that the effects of stress are cumulative.

EFFECTS AND CONSEQUENCES OF OCCUPATIONAL STRESS

The effects of occupational stress are multiform and complex in ways analogous to the sources of stress. This results from several causes: firstly, from the fact that stress has both an immediate and a longer-term impact on the worker; secondly, from the dynamic interactions between differing sources of stress both at work and outside the workplace; thirdly, from ways in which the individual differences and susceptibilities described above mitigate or buffer the effects of stress on the individual worker; and finally, from the poorly understood internal process by which stress actually leads to physiological, psychological and behavioural changes.

Much work remains to be done in order to clarify relationships between sources of stress, individual differences and effects on health and well-being. Still, accumulated evidence overwhelmingly shows that individuals who experience any of a wide range of stressful conditions are at increased risk in developing a physical or mental disorder. Moreover, work settings are likely sources of stress for most people because they provide the main context in which society makes demands on them to perform and to relate to a broad range of people in specific ways.

The following discussion is organised according to the following major categories of stress effects: immediate physiological, psychological and behavioural effects; long-term medical consequences; long-term psychological consequences; and long-term behavioural consequences.

Immediate physiological, psychological and behavioural effects

When confronted with acute stress, the body's resources are mobilised to help the individual to respond to the threat. The body's emergency response is designed to provide the energy for either a "flight or fight" response. Some of the physiological changes involved in the emergency response were cited in the previously mentioned studies. These include increased blood pressure and heart rate; increased catecholamine (e.g. adrenalin) and cholesterol secretion; dryness of the throat and mouth; deepening of respiration and slowing down of the digestive process. These immediate physiological effects provide the maximum amount of energy to the brain and muscles in the minimum amount of time to prepare the body to cope with the threat and to restore its equilibrium (homeostasis). Other common physiological effects which are often due to emotional tensions (psychosomatic complaints) are headaches, backaches, muscle cramps, indigestion, sweating, frequent urination and sleep disturbances.

While these immediate physiological effects occur regardless of the type of stress (i.e. opportunity to do a more complex job, constraint or demand), the immediate psychological effects depend on the type of stress. Associated with the sources of stress described above, the immediate and short-term psychological effects include anger and aggression, tension, irritability, confusion, anxiety, boredom and fatigue. A concrete example is that of feeling frustrated, tense and bored during temporary machine breakdowns. Moreover, these feelings when prevented from being expressed may show themselves in the above-mentioned psychosomatic complaints. These psychological effects or feelings could lead to certain behavioural effects which include smoking, drug-taking, alcohol consumption, speech difficulties, displays of emotion, impulsive behaviour, taking short-cuts, sick leave, and so on.

Long-term medical consequences

Although the emergency response is an adaptive one, prolonged and repeated activation of the body in this manner could lead to degeneration of the body systems involved (particularly the circulatory system), thereby resulting in disease and ill health. One of the reasons why this degeneration happens is that, although the emergency response is preparing the body for intense muscular exertion, most stress situations do not require such a strong physical response which would use up this energy. In fact, many situations are particularly stressful precisely because there is no immediate way out and the individual is helpless or powerless to change the situation.

One of the most frequently studied medical consequences of

occupational stress is coronary heart disease (CHD). Figure 2 illustrates how occupational stress can contribute to heart disease.

Compelling research evidence exists that calls attention to the need to look in greater detail at the characteristics of particular occupations and CHD. Research is beginning to disprove the myth that managers and executives are the most "at risk" group in terms of susceptibility to CHD. In the United States, the Framingham Heart Study investigated the cardiovascular health of women and men over a 10-year period.[79] The participants in the study included 350 housewives, 387 economically active women and 580 men. The results of the study were as follows:

Working [i.e. economically active] women did not have significantly higher incidence rates of CHD than housewives (8.5 versus 7.1 per cent respectively). However, CHD rates were almost twice as great among women holding clerical jobs (12.0 per cent) as compared to housewives. Compared to non-clerical workers, clerical women developing CHD were more likely to have had a non-supportive boss, limited job mobility and suppressed hostility. In addition, the risks of CHD were greater among working women with children.[80]

Another longer-term medical consequence of occupational stress is peptic ulcers. Some studies have shown that peptic ulcer, and in particular duodenal ulcer, is a disorder in which psychological influences are of the greatest importance. However, these studies seem to be limited to male subjects and to such occupations as air traffic controller, foreman engineer and business executive. Findings show that foremen suffered from peptic ulcers more frequently than did craftsmen and executives. Again the data disproved the widely held idea that ulcers are unusually frequent among executives. The incidence of peptic ulcers among economically active women remains a neglected area of research.

Other medical consequences of stress include hypertension, chronic insomnia and physical exhaustion.

Long-term psychological consequences

One of the long-term psychological consequences of occupational stress is neurosis. Neurosis refers to any psychological or mental illness, or to any disability which appears to have a psychological cause or partial cause. It includes chronic states of anxiety, depression, obsession, hysteria or psychosis. Early studies on neurosis among men and women showed that circumstances which were associated with above average incidence of neurosis included working over 75 hours per week; restricted social contact, recreation or leisure interests; marriage with home responsibilities among women, and separation and widowhood among men; work disliked or found boring; sedentary work; work requiring skill inappropriate to the worker's intelligence; work requiring constant attention, especially if offering very limited scope for initiative or technical responsibility; work programmes offering little variety; and

Figure 2. Ways in which stress can contribute to heart disease.

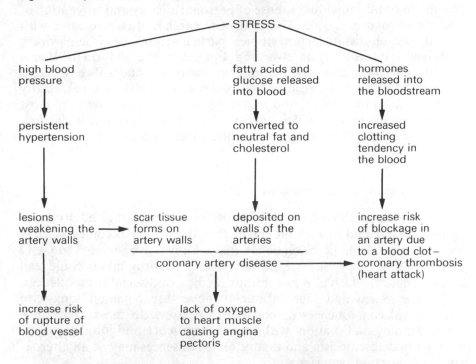

Source: Nicholas McDonald and Mel Doyle: *The stresses of work* (Walton-on-Thames, United Kingdom, Thomas Nelson and Sons, 1981), p. 14.

tasks for which lighting was unsatisfactory.[81] It was found that the most common factors mentioned in connection with these situations were "unsatisfactory working conditions, boredom or monotony, and eyestrain".

While studies on neurosis do not mention data-entry work, the job characteristics most closely associated with neurosis have, in fact, been those described above as typical of data-entry work.

Other long-term psychological consequences which have also been associated with occupational stress are job dissatisfaction, alienation, anomie and apathy. Several previously mentioned studies comparing clerical VDU workers with non-VDU clerical workers and professionals have illustrated that clerical VDU workers who reported high levels of occupational stress also reported the lowest levels of job satisfaction.[82]

Other studies have shown that sources of stress relating to job decision-making latitude and job demands also appear to be related to job dissatisfaction.[83]

Studies on alienation, anomie and apathy usually invoke some aspect of the technological and social organisation of work—

mechanisation, specialisation, hierarchy, discipline or social relations—as a threat to the individual's sense of personal identity and perception of loss of control over the job. This type of research is often associated with job satisfaction-dissatisfaction studies, particularly in cases where work is perceived as intrinsically unrewarding. For example, a study on the effects of mechanisation and automation on industrial and office workers showed that those who executed highly mechanised tasks were especially alienated from their work, and that keypunch operators were the most alienated of all groups of office workers. These workers were also the least satisfied with their job compared to other office workers.[84]

Long-term behavioural consequences

Some short-term behavioural effects, such as smoking and drinking, can be exacerbated to such an extent that the worker becomes a heavy smoker or an alcoholic. Such behaviour is known to be related to CHD and other medical problems. Similarly, occasional drug-taking could lead to dependency, which also has serious medical and social consequences.

Absenteeism and high labour turnover are common long-term behavioural consequences of occupational stress. In most cases, they reflect employee alienation, withdrawal from work and job dissatisfaction. Casual absenteeism and unauthorised absences may be an alternative to separation or resignation.

Because of the physical and mental problems associated with working with machines, data-entry workers appear to be the principal source of worry to personnel departments. For example, in a national survey carried out by the London-based Alfred Marks Bureau, absenteeism and turnover among "data preparation staff" (i.e. data-entry workers) were higher than in any other job category.[85] In addition, vacancies for this type of job were the most difficult to fill.

If workers decide to stay, they may none the less engage in "work-to-rule" behaviour which may undermine organisational effectiveness. Excessive emphasis on compliance with rules and regulations, with frequent recourse to authority and sanctions (the legalities of organisational control), tends in practice to mean that the minimal acceptable standard for quantity and quality becomes the maximal standard. If 60 pages of entered raw text is the standard per week, it is felt that there is no point in exceeding this standard. In other words, what is not covered by the rules is by definition not the responsibility of the worker.

Once such a climate of apathy and low motivation exists, even more formal controls are necessary to deal with the resulting problems of absenteeism, poor-quality work, low productivity, and so forth. Consequently, the initial excessive reliance on formalised rules and regulations, which in itself is a source of stress, leads to more stress as the data-entry worker's job becomes more regimented and constricted. Thus the vicious circle continues. Of course, these problems may also make for a poor industrial relations climate.

Relationship between conditions of work and life outside work

The multiple effects of stress can combine in various ways as they affect each individual, much as the many sources of stress interact to create these effects. What should be kept in mind is that stress is a syndrome: a set of inter-related symptoms which join together to affect many aspects of the worker's life, both at work and at home. Workers who are alienated, frustrated and dissatisfied at work have been shown to have an overall quality of life which reflects this situation. Work "spills over" into personal life. Rather than providing an opportunity for an enriched alternative to working life, leisure reflects and magnifies the problems of work. For example, some American studies have shown that individuals who are strongly alienated from work generally show lower levels of political activity (i.e. they take less part in types of activities that might affect their own living conditions).[86] Moreover, the view that workers may compensate for a monotonous job with stimulating and enriching activities during their free time is gradually being replaced by a better understanding of the strong links between jobs which are circumscribed and repetitious and leisure that is "passive and psychologically unrewarding."[87] Such workers take far less part in organised and goal-oriented activities that require planning and co-operation with others outside work.

Finally, the effects of occupational stress are often "carried over" to affect relationships with families and friends.

Notes

[1] The following recent studies on occupational stress have been published by the ILO: T. M. Fraser: *Human stress, work and job satisfaction*, Occupational Safety and Health Series No. 50 (Geneva, ILO, 1983); L. Levi: *Stress in industry*, Occupational Safety and Health Series No. 51 (Geneva, ILO, 1984).

[2] Working Women Education Fund: *Warning: Health hazards for office workers* (Ohio, 1981), p. 6.

[3] ibid., p. 5; Glen R. Elliott and Carl Eisdorfer (eds.): *Stress and human health: Analysis and implications of research*, a study by the Institute of Medicine, National Academy of Sciences (New York, Springer Publishing Co., 1982), pp. 149–154.

[4] See, for example, Susan E. Jackson and Christina Maslach: "After-effects of job-related stress: Families as victims", in *Journal of Occupational Behaviour* (Chichester, United Kingdom), Jan. 1982, pp. 63–77; Elliott Liebow: *Stress and the work environment*, Panel presentation at OSHA New Directions Conference, Dec. 1980, Washington, DC, cited in Working Women Education Fund: *Warning: Health hazards . . .*, op. cit., p. 7.

[5] Bertil Gardell: "Stress research and its implications: Sweden", in *Proceedings of the Thirty-third Annual Meeting of the Industrial Relations Research Association* (IRRA), Denver, Colorado, 5–7 Sep. 1980, pp. 271–272.

[6] Joe M. Wiley: "Fitting in that extra workload", in *Datamation*, July 1976, pp. 65–68.

[7] Working Women Education Fund: *Warning: Health hazards . . .*, op. cit., p. 12.

[8] Howard Karten: "For only 6% hike in salaries, bank gains 18% throughout", in *Computerworld*, 8 Oct. 1979, pp. 45 and 47.

[9] Introducing new office technology, IDS Study 252, Oct. 1981; *Labour Research*, Nov. 1983, p. 277.

[10] David A. Buchanan and David Boddy: "Advanced technology and the quality of working life: The effects of word processing on video typists", in *Journal of Occupational Psychology* (Leicester, United Kingdom), 1982, No.1, pp. 1–11.

[11] Gunn Johansson: "Psychoneuroendocrine reactions to mechanised and computerised work routines", in Colin Mackay and Tom Cox (eds.): *Response to stress: Occupational aspects* (Guildford, United Kingdom, IPC Science and Technology Press, 1979), pp. 142–149; Gunn Johansson and Gunnar Aronsson: *Stress reactions in computerised administrative work* (Stockholm, University of Stockholm, Department of Psychology, 1980), reprinted in *Journal of Occupational Behaviour*, July 1984, pp. 159–181.

[12] Johansson and Aronsson: *Stress reactions . . .* , op. cit., p. 40.

[13] ibid.; Gunn. Johansson et al.: "Social, physiological and neuroendocrine stress reactions in highly mechanised work", in *Ergonomics*, Vol. 21, 1978, pp. 583–599.

[14] Johansson and Aronsson: *Stress reactions . . .* , op. cit., p. 41.

[15] ibid.; A. Cakir et al.: *Visual display terminals* (Chichester, United Kingdom, John Wiley, 1979), p. 245.

[16] Barbara S. Brown et al.: "Video display terminals and vision of workers: Summary and overview of a symposium", in *Behaviour and Information Technology* (London and New York), 1982, No. 2, p. 132.

[17] Working Women Education Fund: *Warning: Health hazards . . .* , op. cit., p. 11; Gunilla Bradley: "Computerisation and some psychosocial factors in the work environment", in National Institute for Occupational Safety and Health (NIOSH): *Reducing occupational stress*, Proceedings of a Conference, Westchester Division, New York Hospital—Cornell Medical Center, 10–12 May 1977 (Washington, DC, 1978), p. 37.

[18] Michael J. Smith et al.: *An investigation of health complaints and job stress in video display operations* (Ohio, NIOSH, Division of Biomedical and Behavioural Science, 1981, mimeographed), p. 8; reprinted in *Human Factors*, 1981, 23, pp. 387–400.

[19] S. Binaschi et al.: "Study on subjective symptoma—Notology of fatigue in VDU operators", in E. Grandjean and E. Vigliani (eds.): *Ergonomic aspects of visual display terminals* (London, Taylor and Francis, 1980), pp. 219–225.

[20] See, for example, Jon M. Shepard: *Automation and alienation: A study of office and factory workers* (Cambridge, Massachusetts, MIT Press, 1971).

[21] B. Gardell: *Scandinavian research on stress in working life*, Paper presented to an IRRA Symposium on Stress in Working Life, Denver, Colorado, 5–7 Sep. 1980 (mimeographed), p. 4.

[22] Evelyn Nakano Glenn and Roslyn L. Feldberg: "Degraded and deskilled: The proletarianisation of clerical work", in *Social Problems*, Oct. 1977, p. 57.

[23] J. Richard Hackman and J. Lloyd Suttle (eds.): *Improving life at work: Behavioural science approaches to organisational change* (Santa Monica, California, Goodyear Publishing Co., 1977), p. 105.

[24] See, for example, W. E. Scott: "The behavioural consequences of repetitive task design: Research and theory", in L. L. Cummings and W. E. Scott (eds.): *Readings in organisational behaviour and human performance* (Illinois, Irwin Dorsey, 1969); W. E. Scott: "Activation theory and task design", in *Organizational behaviour and human performance* (New York), 1966, No. 1, pp. 3–30; Marianne Frankenhauser and Gunn Johansson: "On the psychophysiological consequences of understimulation and overstimulation", in Lennart Levi (ed.): *Society, stress and disease*, Vol. 4, *Working life*, (Oxford, Oxford University Press, 1981), pp. 82–89.

[25] A. Zvorikyn: "Automation and some socio-psychological problems of work", in Marie R. Haug and Jacques Dofny (eds.): *Work and technology* (London, Sage Publications, 1977), p. 248.

[26] David Grayson: *Job evaluation and changing technology*, Work Research Unit (WRU) Occasional Paper 23 (London, WRU, 1982), p. 6.

[27] C. W. Blakely: "Word processing in the typing pool and the secretarial environment", in Infotech Ltd.: *Office automation: Invited papers*, Infotech State of the Art Report, Series 8, No. 3 (Maidenhead, United Kingdom, 1980), p. 26.

[28] Robert A. Karasek: "Job demands, job decision latitude and mental strain: Implications for job redesign", in *Administrative Science Quarterly*, June 1979, p. 287; idem: "Job socialisation and job strain: The implications of two related psychosocial mechanisms for job design", in Bertil Gardell and Gunn Johansson (eds.): *Working life: A social science contribution to work reform* (Chichester, John Wiley, 1981), pp. 75–93; Robert L. Kahn: "Work and health: Some psychosocial effects of advanced technology", ibid., pp. 29–31.

²⁹ Karasek: "Job demands, job decision latitude, and mental strain . . . ", op. cit., p. 303.

³⁰ Smith et al., op. cit.

³¹ ibid., p. 7.

³² John Thackray: "White-collar blues", in *Management Today* (London, Haymarket Press), Mar. 1980, p. 98.

³³ Working Women Education Fund: *Warning: Health hazards* . . . , op. cit., p. 15.

³⁴ Bjørn Gustavsen and Gerry Hunnius: *New patterns of work reform: The case of Norway* (Oslo, Universitetsforlaget, 1981), p. 132.

³⁵ See, for example, James S. House and James A. Wells: "Occupational stress, social support and health", in NIOSH: *Reducing occupational stress*, op. cit., pp. 8–29; Cary L. Cooper and Judi Marshall: "Sources of managerial and white-collar stress", in Cary L. Cooper and Roy Payne: *Stress at work* (Chichester, United Kingdom, John Wiley, 1978), pp. 81–105; Roy Payne: "Organisational stress and social support", in Cary L. Cooper and Roy. Payne (eds.): *Current concerns in occupational stress* (Chichester, John Wiley, 1980), pp. 269–298; House and Wells, op. cit.; Robert D. Caplan et al.: *Job demand and worker health: Main effects and occupational differences*, NIOSH Research Report (Washington, DC, United States Department of Health, Education and Welfare, 1975); Robert A. Karasek et al.: "Co-worker and supervisor support as moderators of associations between task characteristics and mental strain", in *Journal of Occupational Behaviour*, Apr. 1982, pp. 181–200; A. Billings and R. Moos: "Work stress and the stress-buffering roles of work and family resources", in *Journal of Occupational Behaviour*, July 1982, pp. 215–232.

³⁶ House and Wells, op. cit., p. 24.

³⁷ Smith et al., op. cit.

³⁸ ibid., p. 7.

³⁹ Johansson and Aronsson, op. cit., pp. 22–24.

⁴⁰ ibid., p. 23.

⁴¹ ibid., p. 39.

⁴² ibid., p. 40.

⁴³ R. Elias, et al.: "Investigations in operators working with CRT display terminals: Relationships between task content and psychophysiological alterations", in Grandjean and Vigliani, op. cit., pp. 211–217.

⁴⁴ ibid., p. 216.

⁴⁵ Canadian Labour Congress Labour Education and Studies Centre: *Towards a more humanised technology: Exploring the impact of video display terminals on the health and working conditions of Canadian office workers* (Ottawa, 1982).

⁴⁶ ibid., p. 62–63.

⁴⁷ ibid., p. 130.

⁴⁸ ibid., pp. 145–146.

⁴⁹ ILO: *The effects of structural changes and technological progress on employment in the public service*, Report III, Joint Committee on the Public Service, Third Session, Geneva, 1983, p. 54.

⁵⁰ B. Garson: *All the livelong day: The meaning and demeaning of routine work* (Harmondsworth, United Kingdom, Penguin Books, 1977), p. 173.

⁵¹ Working Women Education Fund: *Warning: Health hazards* . . . , op. cit., p. 47.

⁵² Bertil Gardell: *Psychosocial aspects of industrial production methods*, Reports from the Department of Psychology, University of Stockholm, Supplement 47 (Stockholm, University of Stockholm, 1979), p. 13.

⁵³ Elliott and Eisdorfer, op. cit., pp. 126–127; Nicholas McDonald and Mel Doyle: *The stresses of work* (Walton-on-Thames, United Kingdom, Thomas Nelson, 1981), pp. 26–27. See also ILO: *Payment by results* (Geneva, 1984).

⁵⁴ Cakir et al., op. cit., p. 235.

⁵⁵ ibid.

⁵⁶ In schematic terms, this dichotomy can be expressed as a contrast between the physiological approach based on the concept of homeostasis (from the Greek *homoios* meaning like or similar and *stasis* meaning position, used to describe the ability to stay the same or in a steady-state condition) and the psychological approach which uses other concepts owing to a lack of cognitive counterpart to the steady state implied by homeostasis. Those familiar with systems theory or control theory would refer to this as "dynamic equilibrium".

⁵⁷ Smith et al., op. cit.

⁵⁸ ibid., p. 9.

⁵⁹ Elias et al., op. cit.

[60] M. Rader and J. Gildsdorf: "Preventing environmental stress in the open office", in *Journal of Systems Management*, Dec. 1981, p. 25; D. Hyslop: "Physical environment in the office", in M. Johnson (ed.): *The changing office environment* (Reston, Virginia, National Business Education Association, 1980), pp. 123–124.

[61] Greg R. Oldham and Daniel J. Brass: "Employee reactions to an open-plan office: A naturally occurring quasi-experiment", in *Administrative Science Quarterly*, June 1979, p. 280; Rader, op. cit.

[62] Wolfgang H. Staehle: *Technological and organisational changes in data-entry jobs*, Case study prepared for the ILO (Berlin, 1980; mimeographed).

[63] Tim Davis: "The influence of the physical environment in offices", in *Academy of Management Review* (Mississippi), Apr. 1984, p. 274.

[64] Oldham and Brass, op. cit., p. 281.

[65] Johansson and Aronsson, op. cit., p. 27.

[66] Roy Payne et al.: "Whither stress research?: An agenda for the 1980s", in *Journal of Occupational Behaviour*, Jan. 1982, p. 141.

[67] Douglas T. Hall: "A model of coping with role conflict: The role behaviour of college-educated women", in *Administrative Science Quarterly*, Dec. 1972, pp. 471–486.

[68] Harold W. Wilensky: "Family life cycle, work and the quality of life: Reflections on the roots of happiness, despair and indifference in modern society", in Bertil Gardell and Gunn Johansson; *Working life: A social science contribution to work reform*, op. cit., p. 244.

[69] Edwin E. Ghiselli and Clarence W. Brown: *Personnel and industrial psychology* (New York, McGraw-Hill, 2nd ed., 1955), p. 204.

[70] See, for example, M. Friedman: *Pathogenesis of coronary artery disease* (New York, McGraw-Hill, 1969); M. Friedman and R. H. Rosenman; *Type A behaviour and your heart* (New York, Knopf, 1974); Elliott and Eisdorfer, op. cit., pp. 64–67, 86.

[71] Caplan et al., op. cit.

[72] V. Vroom: "Some personality determinants of the effects of participation", in *Journal of Abnormal and Social Psychology*, 1959, No. 59, pp. 322–327, cited in Marvin D. Dunnette (ed.): *Handbook of industrial and organisational psychology* (Chicago, Rand McNally College Publishing Co., 1976), p. 579.

[73] S. Asch: "Effects of group pressure upon modification and distortion of judgments", in H. Guetzkow (ed.): *Groups, leadership and men* (Pittsburgh, Carnegie Press, 1951), pp. 177–190, cited in Dunnette, op. cit., p. 579.

[74] McClelland, et al.: *The achievement motive* (New York, Appleton-Century-Crofts, 1953); D. McClelland (ed.): *Studies in motivation* (New York, Appleton-Century-Crofts, 1955).

[75] See, for example, S. Seashore: *Group cohesiveness in the industrial work group* (Ann Arbor, Michigan, University of Michigan, Institute for Social Research, 1954); E. Mayo: *The human problems of an industrial civilisation* (New York, Macmillan, 1933); and S. Schacter: *The psychology of affiliation* (Palo Alto, California, Stanford University Press, 1959).

[76] R. Dubin et al.: "Central life interests and organisational commitment of blue-collar and clerical workers", in *Administrative Science Quarterly*, Sep. 1975, pp. 411–421.

[77] Bertil Gardell: "Stress research and its implications: Sweden", op. cit., p. 269.

[78] Walter Rohmert and Holger Luczak: "Stress, work and productivity", in Vernon Hamilton and David M. Warburton (eds.): *Human stress and cognition* (Chichester, United Kingdom, John Wiley, 1979), p. 348.

[79] Suzanne G. Haynes and Manning Feinleib: "Women, work and coronary heart disease: Prospective findings from the Framingham Heart Study" in *American Journal of Public Health* (Washington, DC), Feb. 1980, pp. 133–141; Suzanne G. Haynes et al.: "The relationship of psychosocial factors to coronary heart disease in the Framingham Study: III. Eight-year incidence of coronary heart disease", in *American Journal of Epidemiology* (Baltimore, Maryland), 1980, No. 1, pp. 37–57.

[80] Suzanne G. Haynes and Manning Feinleib: *Clerical work and coronary heart disease in women: Prospective studies from the Framingham Study*, Paper presented at the NIOSH Conference on Occupational Health Issues affecting Clerical/Secretarial Personnel, Cincinnati, Ohio, 21–24 July 1981 (mimeographed), p. 2.

[81] R. Fraser: *The incidence of neurosis among factory workers*, IHRB Report No. 90 (London, HMSO, 1947), cited in Hywel Murrell: *Work stress and mental strain: A review of some of the literature*, Work Research Unit Occasional Paper No. 6 (London, United Kingdom Department of Employment, 1978; mimeographed), p. 21.

[82] See, for example, Elias et al., op. cit.

[83] Karasek: "Job socialisation and job strain . . . ," op. cit., p. 85.

[84] Shepard, op. cit.

[85] Andrew Thomas: "Operators are bored and troubled by office technology, says report", in *Computer Weekly*, 11 Feb. 1982, p. 13, with reference to Alfred Marks Bureau, Statistical Services Division: *The machine dream: A report on the experience and expectations of companies employing full-time machine operators to improve office productivity* (London, n.d.).

[86] H. Sheppard and N. Herrick: *Where have all the robots gone?* (New York, Free Press, 1971), pp. 86–93.

[87] Elliott and Eisdorfer, op. cit., pp. 134–135; Karasek: "Job socialisation and job strain . . .", op. cit., pp. 75–94.

THE POTENTIAL TO IMPROVE DATA-ENTRY WORK

5

INTRODUCTION

The preceding chapters have presented some theoretical and applied studies which show that the data-entry worker is low paid, and has a poor quality of working life and few opportunities for professional development or advancement. The introduction of mechanised technologies in these jobs has exacerbated old problems and added new ones. Many mechanised data-entry jobs are monitored and paced by machines, while many workers are exposed to extra physical and mental strain as a result of increased work pace and workload, and VDU-related problems. However, this is a *choice*, not an inevitable result of the technology. It is increasingly evident that there is no inherent reason why the introduction of word processing should lead to a reduction in job satisfaction or quality of working life. In many cases, the effects on working conditions depend as much on the way in which work is organised as on the technology itself.[1]

The suggestions given below for improving data-entry work are divided into five sections. The first section raises the possibility that data-entry work itself can be rapidly eliminated through technological progress, thereby obviating the need for measures to improve data-entry jobs; this, however, does not prove to be the case. The next three sections, therefore, discuss the content of possible improvements relating to the physical working environment, equipment and office layout; to full-time data-entry work; and to work restructuring and work design. A final section covers the possible roles of governments, employers and workers and their organisations, as well as other key participants in the process of improvement.

ALTERNATIVES TO KEYBOARD-BASED DATA ENTRY

Some observers believe that keyboard-based data entry will soon be obsolete. These observers are optimistic about the potential of direct data entry through character recognition (optical character recognition, optical mark recognition, magnetic ink character recognition) or voice recognition. These possibilities are examined below to see if they are indeed viable alternatives to keyboard data entry in the near future.

Character recognition

There are several types of character recognition devices with differing applications. In spite of the diversity of definitions and names for these devices, they have certain common characteristics and limitations.

Character recognition technologies and products have traditionally focused on responding to user needs in very specific situations. These specialised applications can be found where some form of standardised coding is used. For example, *magnetic ink character recognition* (MICR) is a type of character recognition which was developed by and for the banking industry as a means of processing cheques. For example, with the use of MICR a major United States bank handles approximately 160,000 transactions and 500–900 customer account inquiries daily.[2] However, because of its unique characteristics, MICR tends to be restricted to banks and to similar specialised applications. These include airlines, where character recognition is used to read passenger tickets and freight bills, and government and health-care services, where it is used in processing, inter alia, motor vehicle registration, medical insurance claims and social security forms.

Another special type of character recognition is *optical mark recognition* (OMR), common in the retail and distributive trades. The bar codes widely used in department stores, supermarkets and libraries fall into this category. In these cases, a hand-held character recognition device, often called a "wand" or "light pen", is used to scan and convert symbols into electronic impulses to be processed or stored by the computer. With advances in microprocessor and memory technology, these optical scanners or wands can be incorporated at points of sale and in electronic cash registers to allow not only the automatic recording of product price and identification, but also automatic stock control. However, while OMR may be suitable where a small number of fixed categories (i.e. grid-arranged numerically valued marks) are sufficient, it is not an efficient way to code a large or continuous array of values for a large number of variables.[3]

It is evident that character recognition technology has been effective and accepted in these traditional areas of data processing. Also evident is the limitation of these encoding systems: they cannot handle "mainstream" data-entry applications. These systems cannot be used efficiently for entering handwritten information or information which requires interpretation or transposition as it is entered. Successful applications are therefore found in highly specialised situations.

Today, character recognition is being re-examined in connection with the drive towards growth of the electronic office. Many vendors now support the use of *optical character recognition* (OCR) in conjunction with ordinary typewriters or with word-processing systems. In both cases, the justification is that optical character recognition as a peripheral device reduces keyboard time, specifically "double-keying".[4] As implied by this justification, it is significant to note, however, that the major application of optical character recognition is in "reading" existing typed documents.

Except for very specialised situations, it is questionable whether OCR will be used as a viable peripheral data-entry device capable of coping with paperwork in a regular office. Most experts consider OCR peripheral devices or equipment as merely an interim stage along the path towards the universal use of display-based terminals.[5] The refinement and increased flexibility of visual display (or cathode ray tube – CRT) units, coupled with the increased use of distributed data-entry terminals (communicating word processors), will restrict if not supersede the extensive application of OCR in offices. In the future, OCR is likely to be used to handle graphics, electronic mail, fascimile transmission, and the like, and will continue to serve its original role as a reading tool for the blind. However, as an alternative to keyboard-based data entry, it seems unlikely to be viable.

Voice recognition

Voice recognition is a process whereby the keying of data is bypassed through the direct transformation of a spoken command into machine-readable form. However, this form of input is far from being commercially practical at the time of writing this book. Although voice output is an established technology, voice input is immensely more complicated, and there are some very real limitations and problems.[6] Voice recognition systems cannot understand speech impediments or differences in accents and dialects, nor do they have the ability to distinguish the end of one word and the beginning of another. In addition, they experience problems in dealing with the obvious ambiguities posed by the spoken versions of words such as "hear" and "here", or there" and "their". The higher-frequency range of many female voices also causes confusion on the recognition graph. Moreover, voice recognition systems lack the ability that most human beings take for granted: the ability to filter out extraneous noise, such as office background noise, gum-chewing sounds and the frequent interpolations ("hums and ha's") that characterise human speech. If voice input is made via the telephone, another problem is caused by line noises, line switching bumps, echo suppression effects and frequency distortion.

Work has already started on separated words which are somewhat easier to handle than continuous speech. However, the repertoire of computer-recognisable vocabulary is extremely limited. In most cases, the speaker must "train" the system to his particular voice pattern. This training means that the speaker would repeat one word between three and ten times, while being careful to allow a significant pause between each repetition. For example, equipment reportedly using currently available digital filtering and pattern matching techniques can be trained to recognise up to 64 words or phrases, each up to three seconds in length.[7] For speaker-independent systems (i.e. those without preliminary training) current technology limits the vocabulary to between 20 and 40 words, certainly a long way from being a viable replacement for keyboard-based data entry.[8] Moreover, numbers are preferable to words in designing the vocabulary for speaker-independent systems.

Experiments are currently being made on the recognition of continuous speech without the aid of artificial pauses, but with limited vocabulary.[9] Recognition is based on detailed statistical modelling of all the speech processes involved: sentence production, speaker's pronunciation and processing of the speech signal. The difficulty, according to researchers, lies in the number of sentences likely to be made from a particular vocabulary rather than the vocabulary in itself. In spite of the increasing accuracy rate (up to 95 per cent), it still takes approximately four hours of computer time to process just two minutes of speech.

In Japan, voice recognition is one of the major focuses of research. Although written Japanese is extremely complex and partly accounts for the limited application of word-processing systems in Japan as compared with other industrialised countries, the spoken language is phonetically simpler than English. Various large companies are developing voice recognition devices and products.[10] One, for example, has developed a voice recognition device which can handle 150 words with an accuracy factor claimed to be 99 per cent. It is speaker dependent, with the operator storing his voice pattern word for word. Research at another company has also led to the development of an audio-response system designed for banking applications and telephone input. The device is user independent (i.e. the system does not have to be trained to a particular voice) and can recognise 32 words.

In spite of these developments in both Japan and the United States, advances in voice and machine interface are still only in their early stages. The problem lies not only in developing speech recognition systems but also in understanding "natural" language. There is a strong argument which suggests that unravelling the problems of speech recognition and "natural" language go hand-in-hand.[11] However, in order to understand language, it is necessary to break it down into its components; and to break it down effectively, one must be able to understand what is being said in the first place. A researcher in the field of voice recognition since 1956 considers that high performance speech recognition is still in its research stage, and that the critical characteristics of speech have yet to be discovered.[12]

However, as with optical character recognition, voice recognition is effective for specialised applications. These applications relate mostly to "hands busy, eyes busy" situations, such as quality control applications, materials handling or air traffic control. In quality control applications, inspectors' hands are usually fully occupied, and voice entry allows them to enter measurements which they then visually verify through a display unit.[13] In materials handling, voice data entry permits material handlers to use both hands, keep pace with conveyor systems and enter data simultaneously. Voice data entry will eventually be widespread in air traffic control because it gives air traffic controllers mobility and allows them to use their hands and eyes for other tasks. This is an especially crucial freedom because at present, while keying any altitude or flight plan requested by the pilot, the mind and eyes of the controller are not keeping track of the aircraft on the radar scope. However, since accuracy is critical, a "fail safe" training method would be required to ensure that the computer recognised the controller's speech pattern.

In conclusion, we may say that voice data entry is not a viable alternative to keyboard-based data entry. It is not even a replacement for the keypunch, since it cannot compete with the speed (and accuracy) of an intermediate key-entry operator.[14]

The above discussion of alternatives to keyboard-based data entry shows that, while in certain specialised applications there is significant potential, there are no serious prospects for the accomplishment of the bulk of data entry by such means. Keyboard-based data entry can be expected to remain the major mode of data input in offices for the foreseeable future. Moreover, advances in direct data entry would not lead to the immediate replacement of keyboard-based data entry. Even relatively simple and inexpensive new technologies require a considerable time to replace the bulk of existing equipment. For example, while many offices have installed word processors, a significant number still rely on keypunches and electronic typewriters. The number of existing pieces of data-entry equipment is very large and the quantities of data handled continue to grow. It seems quite safe to predict that keyboard-based data entry will still be a widespread task a decade hence, even if some existing data-entry work has been superseded or automated.

IMPROVEMENTS IN PHYSICAL WORKING ENVIRONMENT, EQUIPMENT AND OFFICE LAYOUT

The simplest and most direct improvements that can be made in data-entry jobs relate to the physical working environment, the data-entry equipment and the arrangement or layout of the workplace.

Physical working environment

The desirable characteristics of the data-entry job are the same as those for any office work, except that special attention needs to be paid to those aspects which are particularly helpful in overcoming problems associated with VDU use and other data-entry equipment.

Lighting

Of the classic features of the physical working environment—lighting, noise, and temperature and humidity—lighting is undoubtedly of the greatest importance with respect to VDU workplaces. Generally, the illumination required is lower than in ordinary office work. For data-entry work which requires reading hard copy, the general room illumination level should be between 500 and 700 lux, depending on the quality of the hard copy. However, in some operations, there will be VDU workers doing different tasks, which may be either screen intensive (e.g. dialogue or conversational) or hard copy intensive (e.g. data entry). In such cases, it may be preferable to lower the room illumination level (300–500 lux) to accommodate the needs of the screen-intensive workers. In this case lamps can be used for those tasks (e.g. reading hard copy) requiring more illumination. Moreover, the best possible shielding to safeguard against both direct and reflective glare should be installed; unshielded fluorescent lamps should be avoided. While some operators use ordinary sunglasses to minimise glare, these may pose a long-term hazard to the eyes. Better solutions include dimming the lights, changing the location of the machine, painting or covering the facing wall in a colour and texture that reflects less light, or installing simple partitions, blinds, curtains or shades. Moreover, for many displays, anti-glare screens are either incorporated into the design or are available as optional equipment. In this connection, it must be noted that some anti-glare screens or filters may degrade the character images on the screen.

All VDU operators should have an eye test by a qualified ophthalmologist before commencing VDU work. Any operator already using corrective glasses or contact lenses should be re-tested. All VDU operators should be re-tested periodically (preferably once a year) and any operator complaining of visual fatigue (eye-strain) should be re-tested. In addition to the eye tests, it is also advisable to record in general terms the type of work involved, since this may influence the extent of VDU use, fatigue and stress. Such record keeping would facilitate monitoring the effects of VDU use.

Noise

VDUs are less noisy than conventional typewriters. Noise in VDU workplaces is usually caused by other equipment in the room, such as printers, telecopiers and telephones, or by nearby conversations. However, VDUs are rarely completely silent; many have a cooling fan or transformer which can whir or hum. Even if the level of noise is low, its frequency may be distracting or irritating to some workers who are sensitive to high-frequency noise and to those whose task requires close concentration.

Background noise can be reduced by a well-planned office environment. Before other types of office equipment are installed in VDU workplaces, their noise levels should be carefully considered. Printing facilities should be in a separate room. Sound-absorbing materials should be used in walls, ceiling and partitions, particularly in open-plan offices.

Noise is more of a problem for keypunch machines. Apart from replacing the keypunch machine with other devices that do not use punched cards, such as key-to-disc or key-to-tape, remedial measures can include installing sound-absorbing walls, panels or partitions, or decreasing the number of keypunch machines in a room.

Temperature and humidity

VDU workplaces have a higher thermal loading than ordinary offices. During their operation, VDUs emit heat which is dispersed by means of a fan. Heat problems may arise depending on the power consumption of the equipment, the room lighting and the number of workers in the room. Although not directly influenced by the VDU itself, the humidity at the workplace is an important factor with respect to the comfort of the operator. Static electricity, which can cause skin rashes in some operators and attract dust to the VDU screen, is also influenced by the humidity level. Adequate ventilation and appropriate temperature and humidity controls should be installed. It is advisable, however, to control the causes rather than the effects of a high thermal load. This can often be done by selecting VDUs with low thermal emission, ensuring that the heat emitted by VDUs and other equipment is not directed towards the operator or the neighbouring operators, and seeing to it that the number of VDUs in a room is as small as possible and is distributed evenly over the office area.

Since people differ in their capacities, preferences and tastes, changes in the physical working environment should be discussed and agreed to by everyone who will be affected. A good solution must take individual differences into consideration to the extent possible.

Equipment

Data-entry workers are in constant contact with the equipment which constitutes their work station. This equipment includes VDUs, keyboards, and office furniture such as desks, chairs, foot-rests and manuscript holders.

Much has been written on the design and possible dangers of CRTs or visual display screens. Most manufacturers have attempted to take account of the following problems:

(a) screens which are too small or the wrong colour;

(b) characters which are difficult to read or poorly spaced;

(c) screen flicker;

(d) glare from improper screen angles, inappropriate materials or ineffective shielding; and

(e) brightness and contrast.

This is no guarantee, however, that all manufacturers produce ergonomically correct screens. Therefore, the many screen characteristics should be checked against standards, guide-lines or ergonomic checklists.[15]

Many workers are concerned about the possibility that radiation from the screens will harm them. Because the screens give off relatively low levels of radiation, it is only in the long run that harmful effects can be expected, and even in the long run many experts claim that there is little or no danger. A careful and factual information campaign can help to allay fears, but the results of the more intensive research now under way are required before clear policies or guide-lines can be set.

Until this is done, VDU operators should be protected from possible potential harmful effects. Careful planning of job and office design can help reduce exposure to radiation. Machines may be arranged so that operators are not sitting too close to other machines, since whatever radiation exposure there is will be multiplied by the number of nearby machines. Reasonable rest breaks away from the screen and periods on the machine alternating with other work will also reduce exposure time, as well as minimise eye-strain. Another interim protective measure is frequent careful maintenance checks for leakage by qualified engineers. This is particularly important for older models of VDUs.

Keyboarding and the design of keyboards have been studied in detail by manufacturers and ergonomists alike. Specifications guide-lines or parameters for well-designed keyboards have been developed.[16] These include the following:

(a) keyboard profile and thickness;

(b) the shape, profile and dimensions of the keys;

(c) the size and coding of the key legends;

(d) key force;

(e) provision of tactile and auditory feedback;

(f) security safeguards;

(g) colour and reflection characteristics of keys and keyboards; and

(h) keyboard layout.

Principal recommendations emphasise that—

(a) keyboards should be detached from visual display screens and should be adjustable so that the operator can arrange the unit for comfortable posture and ease of viewing;

(b) the total number of keys should be limited to the most frequently used functions, since too many keys make all of them difficult to use and the keyboard becomes too large;

(c) the layout of the keys should be such that typical operational sequences form a logical arrangement on the keyboard to help reduce errors and to maintain the operator's keying rhythm;

(d) keyboard thickness (i.e. the distance from the base of the keyboard to the "home" or middle row of keys) should not exceed about 30 mm to facilitate achievement of the correct working height.

It is important to remember that, in all VDU workplaces, it is the keyboard which has the greatest influence on the working method. VDU operators spend most of their working time looking at and using the keyboard. Prior to purchase, appropriate ergonomic guide-lines and specifications should be consulted and, to the extent possible, followed.

Certain features of VDUs may pose safety hazards for users. Like some other office equipment, several components of VDUs operate with high voltages. Although these are normally protected, paper-clips, hot drinks or inflammable liquids should not fall or spill into the VDU through ventilation grills. Chemical hazards may arise if plastic components are attacked by the wrong cleaning solvent or if inflammable liquids are ignited by sparking contacts. In addition, since the operator sits close to the VDU, it is advisable to provide some form of protection in the event of CRT breakage. While the risk of such breakage is low in normal office circumstances, VDUs with a metal band stretched around the edges of the CRT face (which would help to hold broken pieces together) should be preferred. Additional protection may be provided by an implosion shield to safeguard against flying fragments from the rear of the tube.

Ergonomically designed office furniture is not only necessary for the operator's comfort, efficiency and safety and health, but also influences organisational effectiveness. Poorly designed furniture is a major contributor to poor posture and the incidence of back strain. Chair and desk height should be adjustable to match the physical characteristics of the operator. The optimum height of chairs is attained with feet flat on the floor and the thighs in a horizontal position. If the operator has problems adopting such a position, a foot-rest should be provided for added support. Chairs should be provided with adjustable backrests for pelvic and lumbar support. Providing adequate desk space or accessible work surfaces and simple holders for source documents would also reduce postural strain.

Numerous guide-lines and recommendations concerning desk and chair height, leg room, work surface and positioning of source documents exist, and these should be consulted before office furniture is bought.[17] However, even adjustable equipment does not compensate for the fatigue and tension caused by the prolonged sitting and concentration required by some VDU tasks.

Office layout

In addition to specific characteristics of the physical working environment and of particular equipment items, the operator's health, comfort and efficiency are affected by the arrangement of the equipment and the overall layout of the workplace.

Lighting, for example, needs to be considered in terms of the position of the operator relative to windows and other light sources. The operator should not sit facing an unshielded window or light source. The proper placing of video display screens so as to eliminate reflection from glare sources is the most effective means of glare control. Therefore, positioning them parallel to windows, as well as parallel to and between light sources, will eliminate or considerably reduce the amount of screen glare. Nor should VDUs directly face a wall, as this prevents the operator from looking at objects at a distance to rest the eyes. Machines which are too close together or crowded into a small work area can create noise and other distractions for nearby workers.

Ventilation sources should not be too close to any worker. An operator should not be positioned between two machines (i.e. facing one with her back to another), particularly at an angle where the fan from one machine is directed at the operator's back.

How all these factors are taken into account will depend on the size of the room, the number of workers in the room, the size and configuration of each data-entry work station, any other work activities carried out in the same room, the presence of filing cabinets or other office equipment, and so on. Two important points, however, should be kept in mind. First, large numbers of workers in the same room tend to lead to layout difficulties even if the room is large enough to avoid overcrowding. A smaller room with fewer distractions is preferred. Second, certain types of equipment (e.g. printers) are often best placed in a separate room.

Problems related to the open-plan office should also be recognised. As mentioned in Chapter 4, the open-plan office can lead to problems related to noise, movement within the office and other distractions, crowding and lack of space.

In the design of VDU workplaces, there cannot, of course, be one single solution which will suit all situations. In some cases, it has proved desirable to provide workers with an opportunity to experience different equipment and configurations on a "realistic preview" basis. If the workers can subsequently have some say in the final choice of equipment, facilities and layout, this can lead to more appropriate choices and designs.

Finally, it should be strongly emphasised that it is the comfort and well-being of the real individual and not that of some "hypothetical" average worker that is the primary concern. No matter how well the hardware and the facilities of the system are designed to meet the requirements of the job, if they do not match the physical characteristics, expectations and needs of those actually performing the task they will result both in worker dissatisfaction and in production inefficiency (e.g. more errors and delays). In such cases, the cost of poor equipment may actually be hidden within the organisation. Operators can usually adapt and make the equipment work—but at a cost. Even if the cost does not lie in reduced performance, it may result in greater effort being expended by the worker. When that effort becomes too great and prolonged over a period of time, the operator risks damage to health.

IMPROVEMENTS TO FULL-TIME DATA-ENTRY WORK

This section is restricted to full-time data-entry jobs. It covers those jobs for which the only major activity carried out by the worker is encoding or inputting data. These jobs are most frequently found in word-processing and keypunching pools or centres.

The first part of this section examines opportunities to improve the content and organisation of work within the data-entry activity itself. It relates these possible improvements to the desirable job characteristics described in Chapter 2. The second part discusses briefly the relevance of certain working time issues, particularly rest pauses and maximum time of VDU use, for full-time data-entry work.

Work organisation and job content

While full-time data-entry jobs consist of one major activity—encoding or inputting data—there may be variations in the way in which the data-entry activity is actually carried out. These variations result from the differences in the tasks that make up the data-entry activity. The tasks, in turn, may differ according to the type of source material the operator is working from and the complexity or clarity of the text to be encoded. The

113

following are examples of different types of source material:

(a) long manuscripts for original typing;

(b) lists of alphanumeric data;

(c) short letters or memoranda;

(d) insertions in standard texts;

(e) amendments or corrections made by the author on previously typed texts.

The complexity of encoding will vary, depending, for example, on whether the task is straight copy typing from legible material, or typing requiring corrections for spelling, deciphering difficult handwriting, complicated formatting, typing of formulas, foreign words, etc. In other words, given that the overall activity of the operator is data entry, how she goes about it or what she actually does to input the data depends on the type and complexity of the material entered.

In some cases, data-entry workers may perform tasks which constitute "boundary" work associated with, but distinct from, encoding. Such work includes preliminary editing before encoding, proof-reading of typed texts for errors, and so on. These tasks relate to the overall structure of the document cycle and entail going beyond the data-entry activity itself. They are therefore covered in the next section. Verification in keypunching, however, is covered in this section because in spite of its name, it is essentially a repetition of the original encoding.

Autonomy, responsibility and control

There are several factors which make it difficult for the full-time data-entry worker to exercise significant discretion in scheduling her work, or in determining the procedures to be used, and therefore to feel responsibility and control on the job. These factors relate to extreme task specialisation and standardisation, the programming of certain functions into the computer, the misuse of computer capacity to monitor work and isolation from other workers, particularly those not performing data-entry work. In addition, the data-entry worker experiences difficulties in understanding the significance of her work and in obtaining appropriate feedback on performance.

Within these constraints, there are few opportunities to enable the data-entry worker to achieve autonomy, responsibility and control on the job. She could be given the responsibility for contacting the authors directly if she has questions concerning the manuscript she is typing. Similarly, authors could inform her directly of any changes to be made. In order to provide her with some control and decision-making on the job, she could be given several "jobs" to do within a reasonable specified time and be allowed to schedule her own work. This would facilitate her "seeing work through to the end" and feeling a sense of achievement after completing a job, which are important elements of job satisfaction for the data-entry worker.

Feedback about performance is also an important aspect of workers' control over the work process. If the worker sees the computer as a machine that reports performance information to the supervisor, who then uses this information to intimidate her, she will perceive a lack of control over her work. Rather than providing performance feedback to the supervisor, it may be better to give this information directly to the data-entry worker on her screen. She could also key the corrections on the letters, memoranda or reports that she originally typed.

Data-entry work is essentially supportive in nature. The data-entry operator's work has an impact on others, she does not necessarily receive credit for it. It is often difficult for her to perceive the importance of her work to the organisation. However, a few steps could be taken which are likely to provide her with some understanding of the significance of her work and a positive feeling of self-esteem. She could be given some information about the report or manuscript she is typing by the supervisor, or preferably by the author. She could also be informed if she is typing final copy. Moreover, authors could express their appreciation to her and to her supervisor when a job is well done.

It is evident that the potential to enhance the data-entry worker's autonomy, responsibility and control on the job is extremely constrained by the narrow definition of the activity itself. The data-entry worker essentially has no responsibility for steps before and after keying the text.

Workload, work intensity and work pace

Data-entry work has been simplified and standardised. It lends itself easily to work measurement and quantifiable output in as much as the number of lines, pages or key-strokes per operator can readily be determined. Increasingly, the operator loses constant control over the pace, scheduling and organisation of her work. The task and machine have been designed so that the operator spends most of her time encoding, while the speed and rhythm of work is uniform and high. These factors lead to problems associated with quantitative overload, work intensity and work pace.

Overload problems can be minimised in several ways. A first step is the setting of realistic production quotas or standards. The establishment of these quotas should be flexible enough to take account of the difficulty of the document to be typed. For example, some documents are poorly handwritten or otherwise difficult to read; some may contain foreign words, equations, or other unfamiliar copy, while others may require complicated formats. In some cases, authors may make frequent changes as the document is being keyed. Production quotas should make allowances for the additional workload on the operator owing to these circumstances.

Proper scheduling can minimise many overload problems. The scheduling of documents to be typed should take account of both unforeseen circumstances (such as machine breakdowns) and regular peak periods. Production planning and scheduling should consider these factors in advance in order to minimise unpredictable and uneven workloads. Scheduling should be done so that any work disruptions caused by machine breakdowns can easily be absorbed during the following work days. With respect to regular peak periods, the work could be staggered so that normal workload and work pace are not greatly changed. However, these scheduling measures cannot be carried out if the word-processing or keypunch supervisor cannot influence overall work schedules.

Data-entry operators should not be required to work at full speed and meet regular production quotas immediately after passing a training course. They should be given the time to become accustomed to the work situation and to gain some self-confidence.

Finally, the workload should be set taking into consideration individual cognitive, physical and perceptual capabilities, and not merely the capabilities of the equipment.

Skills and careers

For full-time data-entry work, the main skill required is typing. In some respects, the word-processing operator's job is less skilled than conventional typing. Little or no paper handling is required, and corrections are comparatively simple to make. This limits possibilities for the use of different skills. However, the job requires more skill than conventional typing in that the word-processing operator has to learn the different codes for formatting, deleting, merging, and so forth. It is in this area that a limited amount of skill variety can be added to the operator's job. She can learn other "menus", functions and facilities of the equipment. Nevertheless, this means that she must also be given a variety of documents which require using these equipment capabilities.

One of the criteria for a good system is that it should be simple enough for the operator to use without extensive training. Consequently, except for learning and using a wider range of the equipment's capacities, there is little that can be done to achieve skill variety. Even these equipment capacities are designed to ensure that the operator spends less time handling paper, correcting mistakes or performing any other tasks, and more time typing. For keypunching, the main skill required is also typing. There is even less scope for skill variety in keypunching than in operating a word-processing machine. Verification does not require any real additional skill since it consists essentially of re-keying the original data for corrections. In short, full-time data-entry work provides extremely limited—if any—opportunities for the use of other skills besides typing.

Few possibilities exist for careers within the data-entry occupation itself. In spite of the large number of occupational titles and fine distinctions among jobs, there are few substantial differences in duties, responsibilities or pay. Seniority usually results in higher pay, but seniority pay does not in itself contribute towards a true career.

For operators, the only possible advancement is to the grade of word-processing supervisor. However, depending on the number of operators per supervisor, this career step may be limited to a few rather than to the majority of word-processing operators. Some may be quite satisfied with limited career opportunities; for those who are more ambitious and who have higher expectations, however, promotion to supervisor may not be a worth-while career goal.

Social support and communication

Communication and social support are critical factors in influencing the worker's reaction and attitudes towards her job and the organisation. Supportive relationships respond to the worker's affiliative needs and can enhance her self-esteem, as well as influencing relationships among fellow workers and between management and workers. Communication and supportive relationships also facilitate co-operation, problem-solving and commitment to organisational goals. In addition, empirical studies have shown that social support mitigates or buffers the deleterious effects of work stress. However, the nature of the task, the organisational control system, close supervision, the office layout, and informal rules and practices may discourage social interaction and supportive relationships in the workplace.

Within the word-processing centre, where data-entry workers spend most of their working day "interacting" with the computer and repeating the same task, communication with fellow workers is highly restricted. The job has been designed so that required interaction (i.e. the necessary interdependence between tasks, particularly the kind which requires direct face-to-face communication) is minimal, if not non-existent. For work purposes, the required interaction is often limited to the supervisor who allocates and co-ordinates the work. In such situations, there are few ways to encourage communication and supportive relationships.

However, the supervisor has a key role in influencing the kind of atmosphere in which work is carried out. There is little doubt that when the technology requires repetitive and intrinsically unsatisfying work, the supervisor who understands her workers' attitudes, who listens to what they like and dislike about the job and who encourages informal ways of increasing co-operation, job involvement and personalised relationships can to an extent counteract or minimise the negative effects of the job.

Studies have shown that leaders of more productive work groups were those who were in frequent contact with their subordinates, but who did not control them closely.

Techniques or supervisory practices which can lead to destructive individual or inter-group competition (e.g. posting of individual or group daily performance records) should be avoided. Individuals or groups should not be put in a "win or lose" situation where they are competing for some scarce organisational reward. Instead, pooling resources and team-work to maximise the word-processing centre's effectiveness should be emphasised. The supervisor could also discuss work problems with the operators, while encouraging them to suggest changes which could improve the centre's efficiency and effectiveness.

In other words, the supervisor has a key role in influencing the operators' feeling of dignity and responsibility, as well as the atmosphere or "organisational climate" in which work is carried out. Because of the key role played by the immediate supervisor, an effort should be made to provide special training for those who occupy this often-ignored linking position between worker and management.

In addition, direct contact with authors and proof-readers not only widens the operator's perspectives on the work situation and improves her understanding of what is demanded, but also enhances social interaction and mutual empathy.

Computerised systems result in the isolation of individual operators to a greater extent than traditional non-automated processes. This isolation at a fixed work-station greatly reduces social interaction, which has traditionally been one of the major benefits of clerical office work. It is well established that the social support of fellow workers is an important buffer in controlling the health consequences of occupational stress. With the use of VDUs, it is often not possible to interact socially during the task activity. Therefore, social interaction during non-work periods should be encouraged and enhanced. This could be accomplished by providing rest pause facilities close to the work areas and by allowing groups of workers to take a break together.

Working time

With full-time data-entry work, two working time issues are particularly important: rest pauses and maximum hours of work.

Rest pauses

Rest pauses or work breaks are necessary to prevent or counteract the negative effects of physical and mental fatigue. It is now well established that VDU operators experience visual, muscular and psychological fatigue. Although most studies mention the need for frequent rest pauses, only a few make specific recommendations.[18] For example, a 1981 study by NIOSH in the United States recommends that a 15-minute rest pause should be taken after two hours of continuous VDU work for operators under moderate visual demands and/or workload. For those VDU operators under high visual demands, high workload and/or those engaged in repetitive work tasks, a 15-minute rest pause should be taken after one hour of continuous VDU work.[19]

It is the recovery value of a rest pause that is important and not the duration of periods of real or apparent inactivity. Thus, for most VDU workers and particularly for data-entry workers, periods of inactivity such as prolonged system response time and machine breakdown do not constitute a rest pause. Frequent rest pauses which are taken before the onset of fatigue are more effective than longer but less frequent ones.

Finally, rest pauses should not themselves be a source of stress. To the extent possible, data-entry workers should be given some leeway in deciding when to take their rest pauses.

Maximum hours of VDU work

Maximum hours of VDU operation are specified in some technology agreements and legislation, or have been adopted as part of some enterprise-level personnel policies. Various research reports justify or recommend such maxima. The maximum number of hours usually varies from two to four. However, a maximum time of VDU operation implies either that other tasks must be found for the operators or that they must have part-time jobs. Maximum hours of VDU work could lead to the redesign of work of which the data-entry task is just part of a more complex and interesting job. This possibility is discussed in the following section.

IMPROVEMENTS THROUGH RECOMBINATION OF TASKS AND WORK DESIGN

As is apparent in the previous section, there are few options for improvement if the worker's job is limited to full-time data-entry work. This section examines possibilities for making more significant improvements in data-entry jobs through recombining tasks and work design. Essentially, this entails going beyond the data-entry task to see how tasks closely associated with data input, such as editing and proof-reading, may be added to the data-entry task. It also includes combining a range of different activities and responsibilities with the data-entry task. For example, an operator or a group of operators (a team) can be assigned to specific authors, clients or customers.

As in the previous section, these improvements will be analysed in terms of their contribution to the following desirable job characteristics: autonomy, responsibility and control; workload, work intensity and work pace; skills and careers; and social support and communication. Designing jobs with these characteristics will not only reduce the causes of occupational stress but will also result in increased job satisfaction and improved efficiency.

Work organisation and job content

Autonomy, responsibility and control

Data-entry workers are found near the bottom of the occupational hierarchy. While their task is extremely well defined, it is rarely accompanied by any real responsibilities or opportunities to take initiatives and make decisions. This section explores some possible steps which could allow data-entry workers some responsibility and discretion. While the possibilities are still limited, the close relationship between responsibility and the status, self-image and dignity of data-entry workers demands special efforts.

Within word-processing centres, operators could be given some degree of responsibility by allowing them to edit and proof-read their work, to contact authors directly and to have some flexibility in scheduling their work. Some of these steps are similar to those mentioned in the previous section on full-time data-entry work. However, the steps mentioned here require an examination of the entire scheduling and procedures of document production so that opportunities can be found which substantially increase flexibility and provide opportunities for greater autonomy on the part of operators.

Although it is rarely necessary to centralise all data input, it may often be necessary to centralise some of it. Studies have shown wide variations in the responses of operators from one system to another. In some systems the operators are apathetic, alienated and dissatisfied, while in others they have a sense of commitment to the system and enjoy their work. The difference appears to derive from the fact that the latter group have responsibility for the integrity of the data in the system and serve as experts on it for potential users. In other words, these operators are more than just data input clerks; they are often involved in the quality of service that the system provides for its users.

One of the most important work design principles is that the computer system should serve some purpose for the worker keying the data.[20] Efforts must be made to ensure that each worker deals with output as well as input. Terminal use should involve two-way communication, and the other worker should have other tasks which necessitate access to the computer's data base (e.g. dealing with customers' queries). This output requirement has been shown to serve the important psychological function of enabling the worker to experience control over her job. Moreover, it enables her to relate what she enters to what she receives. This may not necessarily mean the same information; what is important is that she knows and understands the relationship. For example, a bank teller may enter details of one customer but may need output for another customer whose details she did not enter. The act of requiring information gives meaning to the act of entering information, as well as clarifying the consequences of poor data-entry. If this relationship is not clear, data-entry can be perceived as meaningless "machine-feeding" and the quality of input can be regarded as trivial.

In situations where a group of workers is given a broad spectrum of duties related to a major area of work (e.g. responsibility for answering queries or updating forms for a group of customers), they have a considerably higher level of responsibility. Although they perform a number of routine duties associated with the input of information to the computer, they also undertake some activities associated with dealing with customers and handling customer queries, which are more demanding and require the use of judgement. In some cases, work group members are made responsible for a greater degree of planning. This may include, for example, arranging the work rota, scheduling the work, and deciding on work patterns and the timing of rest breaks. Thus workers may often handle problems at their own level without having to consult management, thereby deriving a sense of achievement from their work.

Workload, work intensity and work pace

Many of the opportunities for improving full-time data-entry work, as already discussed, also apply. These include, for example, the setting of realistic production quotas or standards, proper scheduling, and providing adjustment periods for newly trained VDU operators.

Extreme functional specialisation[21] is often accompanied by the tendency to accelerate and to increase production standards. When varied tasks or functions are combined to create a more demanding and complex job, this tendency is minimised or prevented. Moreover, the mixture of tasks allows the worker greater flexibility in allocating her time and determining her work pace. For example, the worker can postpone her filing if it happens that some document needs to be typed and keyed urgently. In addition, a worker with a varied job has other tasks to do in case of computer breakdowns.

When the computer system is used to design varied and more responsible jobs, it is easier to make data entry a part of the process of generating the data. For example, in banking it is possible to record the details of withdrawals or credits in computer-compatible form at the same time as the clerk is dealing with the customer. This means that entering data only once is not only more efficient but is also less likely to result in problems of workload, work intensity and work pace. Moreover, it has the additional advantage that data-entry is just an incidental part of a more interesting and meaningful process.

Skills and careers

Various activities can be combined with data-entry in order to provide opportunities for the operators to use skills other than simple typing or encoding.

Some offices have large word-processing centres, where the operators are grouped together under a supervisor. There may also be proof-readers in the same area or in adjacent offices. In such an arrangement, the activities which are easiest to combine with data-entry are editing and proof-reading. The addition of these activities requires the worker to have a good understanding of punctuation rules and knowledge of spelling, a good vocabulary related to the specific business operation and some general idea of the content of the report, letter or memorandum that she is working on. In this case, improvements in the opportunities to use skills do not necessarily entail any radical change beyond the word-processing centre.

The use of present skills can also be encouraged by allowing word-processing operators to interchange jobs on a regular basis with administrative support secretaries. Word-processing operators who were previously secretaries can thus maintain the skills they have developed. For other operators, this means an opportunity to learn additional skills such as those required to establish and maintain a filing system, to operate other office equipment, and to schedule and make administrative arrangements for meetings. They also learn to sort and route mail and other documents to appropriate people. While these are relatively simple skills, they allow the worker to get a better understanding of the office.

In some cases, the traditional office arrangement is preferable to a word-processing pool from the point of view of use of skills. A secretary is assigned to a client (i.e. the chief) or to a group of clients. She uses the word-processing machine to assist her in one task, typing, while at the same time performing a variety of secretarial duties as a part of her job.

A different form of work organisation eliminates the secretarial job as such. In it, a group of workers is given overall responsibility, for example, for all work relating to a group of customers on a geographical or alphabetical basis. This generally means that the members of the group are delegated duties which are often thought to be of a technical or senior clerical nature. Since they are required to process the work, deal with any customer queries, maintain customer contact, and so on, such workers are multi-skilled. In this case, the data-entry work itself is often distributed among all workers and forms a small part of each job. Word-processing equipment is merely a tool used part of the time, and even then "dialogue" functions (i.e. interrogation of data bases to look up and modify records, etc.) are more important than data entry as such.

Extending the boundaries of the operator's responsibilities by adding other duties naturally associated with encoding, such as editing and proof-reading, could open up further career opportunities. After attaining a certain level of proficiency in editing and proof-reading, some operators could be provided with the opportunity to enter the career path of proof-reader and editor. This means that two career streams or paths might be open to a word-processing operator. She could move upwards within either the data-entry operator or the proof-reader/editor career structure.

Allowing word-processing operators to interchange jobs regularly with administrative support secretaries could also provide them with more career opportunities. Apart from the career path leading to word-processing supervisor, they could then also move within the career structure for administrative support secretaries.

In more traditional office arrangements, where the secretary carries out the usual office tasks and activities, the normal career step leading to "executive" secretary could be followed. However, this has its own problems in that her promotion could be dependent on her chief's advancement. In some cases, she could be given the necessary responsibilities so that she could be upgraded to administrative assistant or administrative officer.

In situations where a worker or a group of workers is given overall responsibility, for example, for all work related to a group of customers, more career opportunities are open. Multi-skilled work provides possibilities for the worker to be adept at all or several jobs for which she or her group is responsible. Depending on the type of work and different skills required, this can open up a wider range of career patterns.

Each career opportunity implies a need for the worker to acquire the necessary new skills through training and experience. For example, to be able to enter the proof-reader career path, operators should be given the relevant necessary training. Although specific skills relating to keyboarding, machine operation, filing, and so on, are important, they are not sufficient if career opportunities outside data-entry or word-processing are to be provided. Training should move beyond low-level, task-specific skills to providing a broader understanding of the systems and procedures used in the office. Training programmes should focus not only on the new equipment itself but also on its relationship to the worker's role and the workflow in the organisation as a whole. Moreover, if the data-entry worker appreciates the contribution which her particular piece of equipment makes to the overall function of an office, she may learn to exploit the technology further and to broaden her own responsibilities.[22]

Many women office workers have an interest in the office organisation apart from the practical skills of typing, classification, and so on, that could be the basis of more responsible positions involving training others in the use of office equipment, systems design, sales promotion, customer service, computer programming, and so on. Workers should also be given training to improve their ability in problem-solving, their knowledge of sources of information and the analytical use of data, and communication skills. Moreover, broader-based training will be necessary if workers are to participate in the selection and implementation stages of the new technologies.

There is a need for improvement not only in the content of training but also in its availability. Too often, women are unable or unwilling to participate in training programmes because of family responsibilities. Consequently, training should be carried out during office hours.

Continuous retraining will be necessary to keep up with developments in equipment and office procedures. General training for a career rather than for a specific task should be encouraged. Other training opportunities should be provided in addition to regular on-the-job training programmes. For example, workers who have the ability and interest to learn other skills could be allowed to take time off work to take commercial, vocational or university courses (paid educational leave). This would enable them to take advantage of career and employment opportunities.

Social support and communication

Jobs which require different kinds of tasks also tend to require communication and co-operation among workers. In addition to facilitating co-ordination, such jobs also provide opportunities for understanding the work of others, which can contribute towards a positive organisational climate and good interpersonal relationships. For example, when a group of workers is responsible for a distinct unit of activity consisting of interdependent tasks, it is easier for group members to communicate and to develop group cohesiveness. Face-to-face interaction and each member's comprehension of the range of skills required for the various tasks foster mutual understanding and collaborative relationships.

Improvements similar to those mentioned concerning full-time data entry are also relevant. These relate to the key role of the supervisor, and direct contact with authors and others involved in the work process.

As previously mentioned, office layout, particularly the open-plan office, may actually limit personal interaction and opportunities to develop close friendships at work. While the open-plan office can increase accessibility, it may also decrease the worker's feeling of autonomy, task identity, and feedback from the supervisor and fellow workers. In general, workers prefer privacy to accessibility. Moreover, privacy is often related to satisfaction with work space and job satisfaction. Specific procedures should be undertaken to correct the adverse effects that open-plan offices may have on job characteristics and employees' work effectiveness. For example, screens, partitions or panels may be introduced to give the worker some sense of privacy and personal space or, as previously mentioned, workers should be allowed to participate in the design of their workplace.

Communication and social support are particularly important in the process of change. Steps should be taken to ensure that workers are involved at the outset and remain involved throughout the process of planning, selection, implementation and evaluation of office technology in their workplaces.

Working time

Once tasks are recombined to make more composite jobs of which data entry is one part, it is much easier to improve working-time arrangements. The variations in tasks help to attenuate the physical and mental fatigue often associated with prolonged VDU use. Moreover, changing from one task to another often involves a short pause in work or a break in demand for continuous attention. However, this does not mean that rest pauses should be eliminated, nor does it mean that workers' needs for reasonably flexible working schedules should be ignored.

As previously mentioned, there are rules and personnel policies governing maximum hours of VDU work. Obviously, a job which includes tasks which take the worker away from the VDU screen makes it easier to comply with such rules.

PARTICIPANTS IN THE PROCESS OF CHANGE

The role of government[23]

Some governments around the world have devoted significant resources to issues connected with the quality of the working environment and technological change in general. Recently, however, there has been greater interest in and activity concerning the consequences for administrative and office employees. These governmental resources seem to be concentrated in three areas—

(a) research and dissemination of information about the impact of new technology on the quality of working life;

(b) updating of old labour laws and health and safety standards;

(c) establishment of new legislation and health and safety standards concerned specifically with the quality of working life and technological change.

Research

In terms of research, governments have commissioned studies on these issues, supported research carried out at universities and established research institutes or research programmes related to different problems of working life. In some cases, trade unions have a permanent voice in these research programmes and institutes. National examples from the United States and Western European countries illustrate some of the different forms of government support of research on the quality of working life and new technology.

In the Federal Republic of Germany in 1974, the Ministry of Technology and Research (BMFT) and the Ministry of Labour began a "humanisation programme" which conducts or supports research on the effects of new technology and the humanisation of the work environment. About half of the US$3,000 million annual budget is used for "action research" projects to improve the quality of working life in particular workplaces. These projects must be approved by the local company works council and by a tripartite board consisting of workers', employers' and government representatives. In addition, BMFT also funds basic research on health and safety issues, including the hazards of VDUs and their ergonomic considerations.

In France, the problems arising from new technology and the working environment have been assessed in two major reports, one on the computerisation of society[24] and the other on the impact of micro-electronics.[25] The French Government has also established the Agence nationale pour l'amélioration des conditions de travail (National Agency for the Improvement of Working Conditions—ANACT), which undertakes and sponsors research on, inter alia, work organisation, the working environment, ergonomics and shift work. In addition, it collects and disseminates information in these areas, as well as promoting training activities. Both the research reports and the ANACT have expressed particular concern about the consequences of computerisation for administrative and office workers. Moreover, through its participation in various government bodies, ANACT facilitates consideration of matters relating to working conditions and work organisation in programmes which encourage or use new technologies.

The Governments of both Norway and Sweden have been extremely active in assessing the quality of the working environment and the consequences of computerisation for administrative/office work. In Sweden, some 25 commissions of workers', employers' and government representatives have been formed to investigate the effects of office automation on both employment and working conditions. In addition, the Work Environment Fund was established to give financial support to research on working conditions in the broadest sense. The Government also finances a permanent research institute, the Swedish Centre for

Working Life, to study all aspects of working life problems. In recent years, both groups have worked actively on problems of computerisation in the office sector. They have sponsored basic ergonomic studies of health hazards associated with VDUs, as well as "action research" projects and joint research and education efforts with various trade unions.[26]

In Norway, the Government also supports research projects and research institutes to study working life problems and the effects of computerisation. In 1979, the Ministry of Local Government and Labour appointed a panel of experts to analyse the effects of economic and technological developments on employment and working conditions. Its report, *Employment and working conditions in the 1980s*, was submitted in 1980.[27] This same Ministry has established a special programme to support research projects in these areas. A considerable number of the projects funded have focused on employment issues, the quality of working life and the implications of new technology for office, administrative and service work. Both the Department of Employment and the Department of Work Environment in Norway also finance special projects in those areas.

In addition, the Norwegian Computing Center, which, among other things, carries out research and evaluates policy alternatives for assistance to trade unions on the consequences of new technology, is partly financed by the Government.

The Work Research Institutes, also government funded, have a permanent staff who undertake research both on technical issues related to occupational safety and health at work and on the social and psychological aspects of working life and computerisation.

In Canada, the Task Force on Microelectronics and Employment examined the impact of microelectronics technology on office workers.[28] It issued 30 recommendations designed "to maximise the positive impacts and minimise the negative consequences, thus ensuring a more equitable distribution of burdens and benefits of microelectronics".[29] These recommendations concerned the diffusion of microelectronics, industrial relations, employment, training and education, and quality of working life issues (e.g. health and safety of VDU operators, measurement of work performance and work organisation).

Health and safety standards

Health and safety standards for work with VDUs have often been the subject of trade union negotiations. However, some governments have also proposed or established such standards or regulations. The best examples to date are the Federal Republic of Germany, Japan and Norway.

Safety regulations on the use of VDUs at the workplace were issued in the Federal Republic of Germany by the Occupational Industrial Institute in Hamburg. These regulations, which came into effect on 1 January 1981, list the general standards and VDU design features laid down by the Federal Standards Institute and outline specific guide-lines for each aspect. In addition to stipulating machine design standards and work-station design, they recommend that VDU operators receive regular eye tests and that they are fully informed upon recruitment about the characteristics of VDU work and its ergonomic aspects.

In Norway, the Labour Inspectorate has recommended guide-lines for the use of VDUs at the workplace.[30] Like the regulations of the Federal Republic of Germany, they propose both technical standards and rules concerning working time, training and job content. The draft rule in Norway demands that intense work at VDUs shall be limited to four hours a day or 50 per cent of the working day. A break shall be taken every hour. After two hours' work, the operator shall take a longer break, preferably to do other kinds of work. Finally, the suggested rules demand that tasks be designed so that work with terminals is alternated with other types of related work, with the result that the job is integrated and interesting.

In Japan, the Ministry of Labour notifications of 1964 and 1975 include provision of rest pauses of 10–15 minutes for every 60 minutes of work with VDUs.[31]

National legislation

Matters related to the quality and organisation of the working environment in general are covered in some countries by national legislation.[32] In many cases, this legislation reflects a broadening of the traditional definition of health and safety to include the protection of social and psychological health and well-being through workers' participation in the design of jobs and work organisation. Sometimes co-determination by workers and management in the introduction of new technology or other workplace changes are also included in such legislation, either directly or indirectly.

The Norwegian Act respecting Workers' Protection and the Working Environment (1977) provides for minimum standards, as well as for the improvement of all working environments irrespective of the point of departure. The law is unique in that it explicitly requires good job design to strengthen work democracy and improve physical, psychological and social aspects of work. The participation of employees in the introduction of organisational or technological changes in the workplace is also covered. In addition, the Act calls for the creation of an enterprise-level structure or mechanisms and training programmes to enable employees to take an active role in improving their own workplaces.

In Sweden, the legal framework regulating industrial relations and working conditions is provided in the Act respecting Co-determination at Work, put into effect on 1 January 1977, and the Working Environment Act, which came into force on 1 July 1978. The Act respecting Co-determination at Work gives trade unions the right to influence decisions at all levels and consider all questions related to work and the working environment as open for collective bargaining. This Act is therefore the basis for joint decision-making in areas such as personnel policies, work organisation and the use of computers. The Working Environment Act stipulates that equipment, working methods and material should be adapted to people both from a physiological and psychological point of view.

Both the Norwegian and the Swedish Acts are part of a strategy for improvements in which legislation supplements the shop-floor job reform approach. However, while these legislative instruments form the basis for a more thorough change in organisations, they do not attempt to directly specify the changes themselves.

Another legislative example is the Works Constitution Act of 1972 in the Federal Republic of Germany. Section 90 of the Act requires employers to inform the works council in advance of any plans concerning construction and/or changes in manufacturing, office or other facilities. Moreover, Sections 90 and 91 of the Act require that job design, work operations and the working environment take due account of accepted scientific principles regarding a humane approach to work. Moreover, this obligation increases with time as employers are required to make use of the *latest* scientific findings. The onus for putting this statutory provision into effect lies with the owner of the business or the employer. In line with the emphasis in the Federal Republic of Germany on scientific findings, it is not surprising that the Government strongly supports research.

In summary, it is apparent that governments can intervene in various ways in encouraging improvements at the workplace and in providing protection for the worker. They can support basic research into the improvement of quality of working life. While a large amount of information is available concerning various conditions and problems of working life and what action should be taken, technological development is continually changing the workplace and posing new problems or exacerbating old ones. For example, while knowledge concerning mental or socio-psychological problems has been accumulating for quite some time, additional information is necessary to relate them to such recent developments as extensive VDU use. This is particularly true with respect to stress problems of working women.

Governments can also support applied research, enterprise-level experiments, and pilot projects and their evaluation. This kind of experimentation can be particularly important because it can demonstrate means of improvement, in addition to identifying specific problems. At the enterprise level, overcoming the restraints on the introduction of improvements can be as important as knowledge about which improvements are needed.

Most countries are engaging in a variety of activities directed at the development and application of new technologies. This gives governments considerable influence, and therefore the possibility of encouraging consideration of social factors at the same time.

Governments can update occupational safety and health standards, as well as establish new legislation. One important point about legislation concerns its use. Apart from the fact that legislation introduces a set of binding rules, of greater significance might be the point that a government or parliamentary Act is a value declaration. In other words, it gives sanctions to certain points of view and makes others less legitimate.[33]

Finally, it is significant to note that many governments have established institutions which undertake all these means of action—research, updating standards, developing legislation, collecting and disseminating information and developing training programmes.

The role of management

Management has a key role in the complex challenges, problems and constraints brought about by the introduction and implementation of office technology. It influences, if not determines, when to computerise, what equipment to purchase, the strategy for implementation and the resulting organisational and job changes. Obviously, decisions concerning these areas, in turn, profoundly affect the working conditions and quality of working life of data-entry workers.

The development and implementation of a computer-based system is an investment, and the return on this investment depends on the technical success of the system in meeting productivity and technical goals. However, an increasing number of managers are becoming aware that, no matter how good the system may be in technical terms, it can fail to provide the expected returns. Reasons for failure may, therefore, be sought in the behaviour of those who operate and use the system. As previously mentioned, the introduction of data-entry technology—and the organisational decisions that accompany it—affect workers' individual and collective attitudes, their expectations, the nature of their jobs, their perceptions of the enterprise and their work relations. In most cases, the decision to merely change a typing pool to a word-processing pool leads to familiar problems which can pre-empt opportunities for improvements provided by the new technology. Various work organisation configurations could be examined to ensure that, to the extent possible, data-entry work is shared and no one does it full time.

Immediate supervisors

The representative of management in closest contact with data-entry workers is the supervisor. As previously mentioned, the supervisor has a key role in determining the work climate in the word-processing or keypunch centre. She can encourage collaboration among the workers, and facilitate communication and social support. Moreover, since the supervisor is the first recipient of reasoned criticism from the workforce, she could bring this to the attention of management and system designers. Of course, it must be understood that supervisors themselves are in a precarious position and are also expected to meet particular demands.

Personnel management

Personnel managers and personnel policy determine to a large extent the conditions of work of data-entry workers described in Chapters 2 and 3. The points made in the first part of this chapter are in many cases appropriate for inclusion in personnel policies and practices. Without going over these important points again, a few additional points are made below about the ways personnel management, policies and practices can affect data-entry workers.

Personnel selection and recruitment attempt to match the characteristics of the worker and the characteristics of the job. Various devices and procedures have been developed to assure this congruence. In most cases, they achieve what they are intended to do; but as actually applied, they sometimes encourage practices that are inconsistent with attaining high congruence between people and jobs. For example, the mere availability of tests that place candidates for a position in order of merit can result in routinely selecting candidates who score highest on these tests. While this provides excellent insurance that jobs will not be filled by people incapable of doing them, a frequent side-effect is that a substantial number of people turn out to be overqualified for the work they are assigned to do.

Job evaluation methods also become more important in the light of technological change. The urgency to re-examine job evaluation schemes because of new technology will depend on several factors such as the pace and extent of its introduction, effects on work organisation and job redesign, and required skills. In most cases, there may be signs that a scheme is beginning to become less appropriate. For example, it may be more relevant to describe the work of groups which have collective responsibility than to define individual tasks. Alternatively, there could be a shift in emphasis in some jobs away from conceptual skills to manipulative or mechanical skills. Unfortunately, most existing job evaluation schemes take the current organisation of work as a basic and continuing assumption, which can cause problems when changes in work structures are proposed or implemented. Enterprises will therefore be faced with the task of updating existing job evaluation schemes. Factors and weightings should be re-examined to reflect their appropriateness with respect to the significant characteristics of the jobs concerned.

An important role of personnel management during the implementation phase of new technology is the "protection" of the operators. During this phase, personnel management may find that while the operators are still learning, the "clients" of the system are making excessive demands upon them. At a time when the operators are experiencing doubts about their ability to handle the equipment, such additional pressure can result in negative reactions.

In many enterprises, there are ongoing programmes of organisation development, human resources development, and so on. In most cases, personnel managers have particular responsibilities concerning such programmes. However, there is sometimes a tendency to leave out the lower categories of personnel. This is a dangerous omission, because the most important improvements in data-entry work require at least minor organisational improvements. In fact, personnel management could encourage operator involvement during all the stages of computerisation.

The role of trade unions

Trade unions have consistently sought a very active role concerning the impact of automation and computerisation. As early as 1956, for example, the Trades Union Congress (TUC) in the United Kingdom declared "that the effect of mechanisation on clerical employees might be greater than on manual workers".[34] Since then, trade unions have been deeply involved in investigating office mechanisation and automation, particularly with respect to VDUs. Their usual attitude is not to oppose new technology but to press for the adoption of measures which ensure the best possible conditions for their members. They have quickly recognised that the increasing impact of technological development can be neither ignored nor easily reversed. Instead, they have concentrated on researching the effects of microelectronics on jobs, laying down guidelines to enable their members to come to terms with the predicted changes, expanding trade union education programmes, negotiating technology agreements and participating in formulation of national technology policies. In this connection, trade unions have provided a wealth of reports, papers, books and recommendations.[35]

Trade unions concentrated their early efforts on the effects of automation and computerisation on employment security and pay. Concern about the effects of VDUs on health stimulated interest in occupational safety and health, the working environment and rest pauses, and other working time issues. Current trade union demands go beyond these aspects to include work organisation. This is based on a new trade union strategy—

There is . . . a discernible trend towards union intervention in the process of technological change at an earlier stage in the decision-making process. Whereas unions have always had to react to change and negotiate the effects of changes, they are now in general seeking to influence the direction of that change itself so as to better insure that the effects upon their members can be influenced.[36]

However, the inclusion of work organisation issues in trade union positions and demands has raised a number of delicate issues—

The trade unions consider that it is difficult for them to establish a reasonable relationship to such changes under the traditional legal superstructure, which gives management control over issues of work organisation. Any development, any contribution from the employees would be outside the domain where they have any statutory authority or possibilities of safeguarding any progress.[37]

In many countries, legislation on workers' participation or new bargaining developments has opened up ways to overcome these problems. Thus, according to FIET—

Trade union strategies . . . must therefore aim to make computerisation decisions the result of negotiation between management and unions and indeed to ensure that the whole process, once this decision is made, becomes a joint undertaking with joint control at all levels of the enterprise.[38]

In some countries, such as the Federal Republic of Germany, Norway and Sweden, legislation has made it possible for trade unions to achieve this aim by giving union members representation on company boards of directors or other management decision-making bodies. For example, under the Acts concerning co-determination, trade unions have the right to participate in management decisions concerning the development and introduction of new processes and equipment.

Trade union action is in some countries limited by very weak trade union membership among data-entry workers. In the United States, for example, only 11 per cent of such workers belong to trade unions.[39] However, even in these cases trade union demands and collective agreements may have an influence beyond the trade union membership itself, by becoming a model for good practice.

The content of trade union demands may be seen from trade union policy statements, model technology agreements, checklists and guidelines for negotiation, various trade union action programmes, collective bargaining kits, and trade union training and education programmes. For example, in the United Kingdom, the Association of Professional, Executive, Clerical and Computer Staff has published and circulated widely a model technology agreement which can be the basis for negotiations between unions and employers concerning the introduction of new technology.[40] This model agreement covers aspects such as joint management/union planning and implementation, job loss or redundancy, reductions in the working week and working hours, safety and health, job evaluation, grievance/dispute procedures, training, and access to data to enable workers' representatives to monitor the impact of the changes. Furthermore, the model agreement covers the content of jobs and job satisfaction. Specifically, it advocates that full analysis be carried out, through joint union/management committees, on the effects of new systems on job content and job satisfaction. In addition, jobs should be carefully designed to ensure that routine and monotony are minimised.[41]

In October 1984 the International Trade Union Conference on Visual Display Units, meeting in Geneva, drew up a set of international guide-lines.[42] It was hoped that the guide-lines would serve trade union negotiators involved in collective bargaining and would constitute a common policy of the international trade union organisations in their attempt to influence international standard-setting bodies.

Trade union training and education also reflect trade union demands and recommendations concerning new technology. These can consist of residential courses, briefing seminars for staff representatives, conferences and national level courses. International training activities are also arranged in co-operation among different trade unions. For example, trade unions in Austria, the Federal Republic of Germany, Luxembourg and Switzerland collaborated in conducting training on ergonomics.[43] Subjects covered in these training courses include, among others, participation, planning and control, working conditions, health and safety, job evaluation, wage systems, working environment and group work. New technology and its practical organisational applications will become an increasingly important part of these training activities, and trade unions will develop more training materials in this field. For example, the TUC and the Swedish Union of Social Insurance Employees have recently published training materials entitled "New technology case studies" and "New data", respectively.

In many countries in Europe, such as the Federal Republic of Germany, Norway, Sweden and the United Kingdom, trade unions have obtained government grants to establish training courses, particularly for trade unionists who act as "data shop stewards" or technology committee members.[44] In the Federal Republic of Germany and the United Kingdom training programmes are also subsidised by national ministries of industry, research or technology. In Scandinavia, national working environment funds, which are financed mostly by employers' contributions, are also sources of funding for trade union training courses. In many countries in Western Europe, trade unions make use of national legislation requiring management to pay for the training of shop stewards, safety committee members or local union officers in company time.

However, trade unions "often lack sufficient technical expertise to bargain effectively over complex new technology issues".[45] Consequently, they have developed close relationships with experts and researchers from universities, technical and research institutes, and consulting firms. For example, staff members of the Norwegian Computing Centre and the Swedish Centre for Working Life act as consultants to local trade unions. In the United States, NIOSH has also conducted extensive field investigations concerning VDUs and health hazards at the request of a consortium of trade unions.[46] Moreover, it is significant to note that many computer and electronics firms in Europe are unionised. This means that staff directly involved in the development of new technology also serve as resource persons for fellow union members.

Collective barganing

Trade unions have also expanded the scope of collective bargaining to ensure that technological questions are covered and that the interests of their members are considered at stages when technological decisions can be influenced. In a growing number of countries, technology agreements which deal with the introduction of new technology, particularly of computer-based systems and VDUs, have been negotiated mostly at the initiative of trade unions. These agreements usually cover both procedural and substantive issues.

The procedural issues typically specify—

(a) the commitment of both parties to the introduction of new technology and the satisfactory management of change;

(b) the provision of information by management to trade unions on the introduction of new technology as early as possible, before decisions are taken and when final choices can still be influenced;

(c) the establishment of labour-management committees to discuss, monitor and negotiate changes;

(d) the opportunity for trade unions to elect representatives with specific responsibility for monitoring the introduction of new technology; and

(e) access to outside expertise for trade unions.[47]

In terms of substantive issues, as regulated by these procedures, technology agreements usually cover work redesign, training and retraining, ergonomic standards, work organisation, job evaluation and guarantees against deskilling and downgrading. For example, an agreement might specify the following:

(a) no redundancies to be declared as a result of the introduction of new technologies; staff whose jobs are changed or eliminated should be retrained and given jobs of comparable status;

(b) no increase in the pace of work, control or supervision or reduction in job content as a result of the introduction of new technology;

(c) consideration of job satisfaction in the jobs created or affected by the introduction of new technology;

(d) close regulation of health and safety aspects of working with computerised equipment and VDUs (e.g. the design of the equipment and the working place should conform to ergonomic standards; the amount of time spent working with VDUs should be limited; regular breaks away from the machine should be provided for; and regular medical checks, particularly eye examinations, should be made available);

(e) provision of training, particularly for selected union members. Such training will include an appreciation of the total system, health and safety implications, basic ergonomic principles, etc.; and

(f) a full analysis of the effects of new technology on the existing job evaluation scheme and, if necessary, negotiation of a new job evaluation scheme.[48]

In the United Kingdom, the TUC has developed a "checklist for negotiators" concerning new technology.[49] The following areas, among others, are covered by the checklist:

(a) the principle of technology agreements (e.g. joint management/union decision-making, and scope for trade union action where collective agreements contain status quo provisions);

(b) provision of full and regular information on which the key decisions taken by companies are based;

(c) retraining;

(d) hours of work, with the aim of distributing the benefits of technology;

(e) health and safety;

(f) control over work (e.g. procedures for individual and collective work performance measurement); and

(g) procedures for reviewing progress against objectives set out in new technology agreements.

The Newspaper Guilds in the United States have also developed a *VDT-health collective bargaining kit* which contains guide-lines concerning health and safety issues.[50]

Although most technology agreements that have been negotiated have dealt with the introduction of computer-based systems and the use of VDUs, some agreements take a broader approach to include all types of technological change (e.g. in Norway). In other cases, collective agreements take a more integrated comprehensive approach covering many aspects of change and working conditions, and include as one element clauses regulating new technology. For example, Swedish agreements often take an overall approach covering planning, rationalisation, consultation, training and careers in one and the same context.[51] It is likely that such comprehensive agreements will spread in the near future in some countries. However, they may be more difficult to negotiate compared with proposed agreements which are restricted to specific issues.

Notes

[1] ILO: *Automation, work organisation and occupational stress*, Report, conclusions and working papers of the Meeting of Experts on Automation, Work Organisation, Work Intensity and Occupational Stress (Geneva, 1984).

[2] C. L. Littlefield et al.: *Office and administrative management: Systems analysis, data processing and office services* (Englewood Cliffs, New Jersey, Prentice Hall, 3rd ed., 1970), p. 235.

[3] James C. Taylor: *Fragmented office jobs and the computer* (Geneva, ILO, 1978; mimeographed internal working document; restricted).

[4] B. Streater: "OCR: Beating the keyboard bottleneck", in *Computing Europe*, 26 Oct. 1978, p. 22; Marly Bergerud and Jean Gonzalez: *Word processing: Concepts and careers* (Chicago, John Wiley, 1978), p. 82.

[5] United Kingdom, Department of Industry: *Microprocessor applications: Cases and observations*, Report prepared by the Massachussetts Institute of Technology (London, 1979), p. 71.

[6] Rita Shoor: "Natural speech recognition? Not till '90", in *Computerworld*, 13 Oct. 1980, p. 79; "What's ahead in DP?", in *Computerworld* 12 Jan. 1981, In-Depth/8; Howard A. Karten: "Vocal access system devised", in *Computerworld*, 8 Jan. 1979, p. 47.

[7] "Voice recognition: Today and tomorrow", in *Computerworld*, 9 June 1980, p. 53.

[8] *Computerworld*, 13 Oct. 1980.

[9] *Computerworld*, 9 June 1980, pp. 51 and 53.

[10] R. Garner and M. Coffey: "NEC leads in achievements from Japan", in *Computing Europe*, 4 Mar. 1982, p. 24.

[11] P. Manchester: "Research unties double knot", in *Computing Europe*, 4 Mar. 1982, p. 21.

[12] Garner and Coffey, op. cit.

[13] E. Joseph Simmons: "Voice data entry handles perishable information best", in *Computerworld*, 23 Apr. 1979.

[14] ibid.

[15] See, for example, A. Cakir et al.: *Visual display terminals* (Chichester, United Kingdom, John Wiley, 1980); E. Grandjean and E. Vigliani (eds.): *Ergonomic aspects of visual display terminals* (London, Taylor and Francis, 1980).

[16] See, for example, Cakir et al., op. cit., pp. 122–144; Grandjean and Vigliani, op. cit.; E. Grandjean et al.: "Preferred VDT workstation settings, body posture and physical impairments", in *Applied Ergonomics*, June 1984, pp. 99–104.

[17] See, for example, Cakir et al., op. cit., pp. 159–173; Grandjean and Vigliani, op. cit., pp. 167–195, 277–288; Federal Republic of Germany, Deutscher Institut für Normung: *Safety regulations for display workplaces in the office sector* (IBM internal document; mimeographed; 1980).

[18] United Kingdom, Labour Research Department: *Survey of new technology*, Bargaining Report No. 22 (London, n.d.), p. 14.

[19] Michael J. Smith: *Health issues in VDT work* (Cincinnati, Ohio, NIOSH, n.d.; mimeographed), p. 39.

[20] K. Eason and R. Sell: "Case studies in job design for information processing tasks", in E. N. Corlett and J. Richardson (eds.): *Stress, work design and productivity* (Chichester, United Kingdom, John Wiley, 1981), pp. 195–199.

[21] In this case, functional specialisation implies that a group of people is assigned exclusively to perform a single type of activity such as data entry.

[22] Manpower Services Commission: *Women and Training News* (London), Winter 1980, p. 8.

[23] Parts of this section are based on drafts prepared by Miss Leslie Schneider, currently with the Kennedy School of Government, Harvard University, Cambridge, Massachusetts.

[24] S. Nora and A. Minc: *Informatisation de la société* (Paris, La Documentation française, 1978).

[25] P. Bonelli and A. Fillion: *L'impact de la microélectronique: Préparation du huitième plan, 1981–1985* (Paris, La Documentation française, 1981).

[26] I. Backlund et al.: *KATA Projektet: Kvinnors arbete, teknik och alternativ* [KATA Project: Women's work, technique and alternative] (Stockholm, Arbeitslivscentrum, 1980); B. Göranzon: *Job design and automation in Sweden: Skills and computerisation* (Stockholm, Arbeitslivscentrum, 1983).

[27] *Norges Offentlige Utredninger* (Oslo), 1980: 33, Issue on employment and working conditions in the 1980s.

[28] Labour Canada: *In the chips: Opportunities, people, partnerships* (Ottawa, 1982); Harish C. Jain: "Task Force encourages diffusion of microelectronics in Canada", in *Monthly Labor Review*, Oct. 1983, pp. 25–29.

[29] Jain, op. cit., p. 25.

[30] L. Hjort: *Utkast til forskrifter og veiledning vedrørende: Arbeidsplasser ved skjermterminaler* [Outline for regulations and guide-lines concerning workplaces with VDU terminals] (Oslo, Direktoret for Arbeidstilsynet, 1981).

[31] Hajime Saito et al.: *Work-rest schedules and related problems of key operators dealing with computer input data: Results of a survey on 310 establishments*, Case study prepared for the ILO (Kawasaki, Japan, 1979; mimeographed).

[32] ILO: "Work organisation and the introduction of new technology: A survey of legislation and collective agreements in industrialised countries", in ILO: *Automation, work organisation and occupational stress*, op. cit., pp. 33–72.

[33] Bjørn Gustavsen and Gerry Hunnius: *New patterns of work reform: The case of Norway* (Oslo, Universitetsforlaget, 1981).

[34] G. L. Simons: *Introducing microprocessors* (Manchester, National Computing Centre, 1979), p. 137.

[35] See, for example, Association of Professional, Executive, Clerical and Computer Staff (APEX): *Office technology: The trade union response* (London, 1979); International Federation of Commercial, Clerical and Technical Employees (FIET): *Computers and work – FIET action programme* (Geneva, 1979); C. Jenkins and B. Sherman: *The collapse of work* (London, Eyre Methuen, 1979); Association of Scientific, Technical and Managerial Staffs: *Technological change and collective bargaining*, Discussion document (London, 1980); Confédération française démocratique du Travail: *Les dégâts du progrès* (Paris, 1977); European Trade Union Institute (ETUI): *Collective bargaining in Western Europe 1979–80 and prospects for 1981* (Brussels, 1981); idem: *Redesigning jobs: Western European experiences* (Brussels, 1981); idem: *The impact of microelectronics on employment in Western Europe in the 1980s* (Brussels, 1979); American Federation of Labor-Congress of Industrial Organizations: *Co-operation or conflict: European experiences with technological change at the workplace* (Washington, DC, Department for Professional Employees, 1981).

[36] ETUI: *Collective bargaining in Western Europe . . .*, op. cit., p. 270.

[37] Bertil Gardell and Bjørn Gustavsen: "Work environment research and social change: Current developments in Scandinavia", in *Journal of Occupational Behaviour*, Jan. 1980, p. 11.

[38] FIET: *Conference on computers and work, Velm, Austria, 17–18 November 1978* (mimeographed), p. 16.

[39] Ann Crittendon: "Interest in unionising increases among female office workers", in *New York Times*, 9 July 1979.

[40] APEX: *Automation and the office worker* (London, 1980).

[41] ibid., Clause 7, p. 58.

[42] FIET: *International trade union guidelines on visual display units* (Geneva, 1985).

[43] ETUI: *Redesigning jobs . . .*, op. cit., p. 225.

[44] Steve Early: "Unions and management in Europe seek to ease transition to new technology", in *Transatlantic Perspectives* (Washington, DC, German Marshall Fund of the United States), Feb. 1982, pp. 20–24.

[45] ibid., p. 23.

[46] See, for example, Michael J. Smith et al.: *An investigation of health complaints and job stress in video display operations* (Ohio, NIOSH, 1981).

[47] ETUI: *Collective bargaining in Western Europe . . .*, op. cit., pp. 268–269.

[48] ibid., 269–270.

[49] United Kingdom, Trades Union Congress: *Employment and technology*, Report to the 1979 Congress (London, 1979), pp. 64–71; "United Kingdom: New technology agreements", in *European Industrial Relations Review*, July 1982, pp. 25–27; ETUI: *The impact of microelectronics on employment . . .*, op. cit., pp. 140–151.

[50] United States, Newspaper Guild: *VDT-health collective bargaining kit* (Washington, DC, 1977).

[51] ETUI: *Redesigning jobs . . .*, op. cit., p. 199.

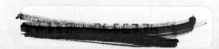